病理学学习指导
（汉英对照）

Pathology
Study Guide in Chinese and English

主 编 何妙侠

Editor-in-chief Miaoxia He

上海科学技术出版社

图书在版编目（CIP）数据

病理学学习指导：汉英对照 / 何妙侠主编. -- 上
海：上海科学技术出版社，2023.9（2025.1重印）
ISBN 978-7-5478-6249-0

Ⅰ. ①病… Ⅱ. ①何… Ⅲ. ①病理学－高等学校－教
学参考资料－汉、英 Ⅳ. ①R36

中国国家版本馆CIP数据核字(2023)第125165号

病理学学习指导（汉英对照）

主编　何妙侠

上海世纪出版（集团）有限公司
上 海 科 学 技 术 出 版 社　出版、发行
（上海市闵行区号景路159弄A座9F-10F）
邮政编码201101　www.sstp.cn
上海光扬印务有限公司印刷
开本　787×1092　1/16　印张 16
字数 250千字
2023年9月第 1 版　2025年1月第 2 次印刷
ISBN 978-7-5478-6249-0 / R·2793
定价：80.00元

序 一

　　病理学是研究疾病发生的原因、发生机制、病理变化、发展规律和转归，从而揭示疾病本质的科学。"病理乃医学之本"（As is our pathology, so is our medicine），出自"现代医学之父"威廉·奥斯勒（William Osler），这句话充分肯定了病理学在医学中的重要地位和作用。病理学作为重要和关键的桥梁学科，兼有基础医学和临床医学属性与任务。病理学课程是临床医学及相关专业学生的骨干必修课，链接基础医学课程与临床医学课程。另一方面，病理诊断是疾病诊断的"金标准"，病理医生被誉为"医生的医生"。因此，病理学是每一位医学生学习生涯中较为重要的必修课之一，掌握病理学知识和技能在医疗实践服务中十分重要。

　　掌握解剖学、组织学、生理学、生物化学和微生物学等基础医学知识是学好病理学的前提。医学生从学习病理学阶段便开始全面接触疾病的共性特征（病理学总论）和个性表现（病理学各论），实现从基础课到临床课的重要过渡。病理学专业术语多、形态描述多、复杂机制多、动态变化多、结局转归多。学生既要深刻理解、牢记病变，又要灵活掌握、了解前沿，还要预习必要的临床课程知识，时刻联系临床表现，为今后学好内科、外科、妇科、儿科等临床医学课程打下良好基础。病理学的疾病、病变和并发症术语都有专用英文名称，医学生如能在此阶段学习疾病的基础上，进一步掌握相关名词术语的英文表达，对帮助学生提高医学英文文献阅读能力，进一步播下临床科研的种子，成为高素质医学人才具有重要的意义。

　　《病理学学习指导（汉英对照）》是海军军医大学第一附属医院病理科、病理解剖学教研室在总结多年来八年制医学生病理学课程中英文双语教学的宝贵经

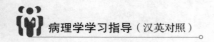

验基础上，由教研室主任何妙侠教授带领学员编撰的辅助学习资料。该学习指导以《病理学》全国统编教材为基础，按照病理学教学大纲要求和八年制病理学课程标准编纂而成。该学习指导既全面涵盖了病理学基本知识点，又重点突出、便于记忆，十分契合学生的学习特点与需求。我认为，这是一本简明扼要，很适合本科生学习病理学课程的实用辅导教材。

祝贺《病理学学习指导（汉英对照）》一书出版！

中国科学院院士

西南医院病理科、病理学教研室

2023 年 7 月

序 二

　　病理学是联系基础医学与临床医学的重要桥梁课,学生在学习病理学阶段开始接触疾病,面临从基础课到临床课的重要过渡。长海医院病理科、病理解剖学教研室一直承担海军军医大学(原第二军医大学)本科生的病理学教学工作。从2010年开始,在临床医学专业八年制本科生病理学课程教学过程中率先推行了中英文双语教学模式,该项工作的开展由校特级优秀教师郑唯强教授牵头实施,并得到了澳大利亚墨尔本大学医学院 William Richard 教授的支持和帮助,现由长海医院病理科主任何妙侠教授主讲完成。经过长海医院病理科、病理解剖学教研室几代人的努力,病理学双语教学课程现已成为海军军医大学本科生的教学特色课程之一,受到学生的充分肯定和热烈欢迎。总结十余年来病理学双语教学的经验与体会,在某些方面双语教学优于纯英语教学,单纯追求纯英语教学会影响学生对病理基础知识的掌握。同时,双语教学形式可以多样化,授课老师可以根据自己的英语表达情况,结合学生的英语基础,采取合适的授课方式,一方面培养学生学习医学英语的兴趣,另一方面则可达到病理学教学的目的,真正体现双语教学的价值。我们从多年的教学实践和与学生的反复互动过程中体会,如果有一本专门针对病理学各章节内容的简易中英文对照学习指导,对帮助学生做好课前预习与课后复习,及时掌握病理学知识和相关词汇,提高双语教学效果大有裨益。应学生的提议和要求,由带教老师编写了《病理学学习指导(汉英对照)》,旨在帮助学生在学习病理学的同时能掌握基本的病理学英语词汇,为进一步学习临床医学知识打好基础,并在一定程度上提高查阅医学英文文献的能力。

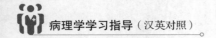

　　《病理学学习指导（汉英对照）》严格按照病理学教学大纲要求和八年制病理学课程标准，以病理学统编教材为基础，突出课程学习重点，并采用双栏双语对照形式编辑，便于学生查阅和记忆，充分彰显实用性和可读性，有望成为一本深受学生喜爱的病理学辅导教材。

　　我衷心祝贺该书的出版并乐为之序。

海军军医大学第一附属医院

病理科主任医师、教授

2023 年 7 月

前　言

　　病理学是研究疾病的病因、发病机制、病理变化、结局及转归的医学基础学科，它是临床医学与基础医学之间的桥梁。病理学教学中涉及众多人体正常组织、器官结构以及人类常见疾病名称、术语、病理变化、临床表现等，是医学生成长过程中必修的重要内容。掌握病理专业术语以及相应英文表述，对帮助学生学好病理、培养临床思维能力，查阅文献等具有很大帮助。我校八年制学员是临床医学专业的精英，学生对知识的接受能力较强，我们对八年制学生进行了中英双语教学，取得了良好的效果。

　　教学过程中，我们发现学生在中英文双语学习中存在的主要障碍是对病理学专业术语的英语表达，为帮助学生尽快掌握常见疾病的病理特征与术语的英文表达，提高病理学双语教学的效果，我们根据多年的教学经验编写了《病理学学习指导（汉英对照）》，主要参照 *Robbins Basic Pathology* 的基本知识点，根据病理学教学大纲要求和课程标准，严格遵守病理学教材的知识要点，同时结合教学过程的授课经验，以病理学教学章节为基础对知识点进行了系统梳理，做到重点突出、条理清楚、易于记忆、中英文表达规范，便于学生在学习过程中能抓住重点，掌握常见病、多发病的基本病理特征，熟悉相应的英文表述，并能做到举一反三，真正体现病理学双语教学在基础医学教育和临床医学教育中的桥梁作用。

　　《病理学学习指导（汉英对照）》的编写参考了我校2016级临床医学八年制学员整理的病理学课堂笔记，在此我代表长海医院病理科、病理解剖学教研室对顾昊煜、何晨、蒋薇、李满平、秦铭、朱光浩等同学的辛勤付出表示衷心感谢！

2023 年 7 月

CONTENTS/ 目录

Introduction to pathology

001

病理学绪论

001

General pathology

007

病理学总论

007

Chapter 1   Adaptation and Injury of Cell and Tissue 009

第1章   细胞和组织的适应与损伤 009

Section 1   Adaptation 009

第1节   适应 009

Section 2   Causes and mechanism of cellular injury 012

第2节   细胞损伤的原因和机制..... 012

Section 3   Reversible injury: Degeneration 014

第3节   可逆性损伤：变性............ 014

Section 4   Irreversible injury: Cell death 018

第4节   不可逆性损伤：细胞死亡 018

Chapter 2   Repair of injury 025

第2章   损伤的修复 025

Section 1   Repair by regeneration 025

第1节   再生性修复 025

Section 2   Repair by fibrinous tissue 030

第2节   纤维性修复 030

Section 3   Healing of wound 031

第3节   伤口愈合 031

Chapter 3   Local Blood Circulation Disorders 033

第3章   局部血液循环障碍 033

Section 1   Hyperemia and Congestion 033

第1节   充血和淤血..................... 033

Section 2　Thrombosis......................036

Section 3　Embolism 040

Section 4　Infarction....................044

Chapter 4　Inflammation 046

Section 1　Conception of inflammation

...................................046

Section 2　Acute inflammation 048

Section 3　Chronic inflammation......055

Chapter 5　Neoplasm....................058

Section 1　Conception of neoplasm

...................................058

Section 2　Morphology of neoplasm

...................................059

Section 3　Tumor nomenclature and

classification 061

Section 4　Tumor growth, invasion, and

metastasis 062

Section 5 & 6　Tumor grading, staging,

and influence on patients

...................................065

Section 7　Comparison of benign and

malignant 066

Section 8　Common tumors.............067

Section 9　Precancerous diseases, dysplasia

and carcinoma *in situ* 069

Section 10　Molecular mechanism of

tumorigenesis 070

Section 11&12　Environmental and

genetic factors of

tumorigenesis 071

第2节　血栓形成................036

第3节　栓塞................040

第4节　梗死................044

第4章　炎症................046

第1节　炎症概述................046

第2节　急性炎症................048

第3节　慢性炎症................055

第5章　肿瘤................058

第1节　肿瘤的概念................058

第2节　肿瘤的形态................059

第3节　肿瘤的命名和分类............061

第4节　肿瘤的生长、扩散与

转移................062

第5&6节　肿瘤分级与分期　肿瘤对

机体的影响................065

第7节　良性肿瘤与恶性肿瘤........066

第8节　常见肿瘤................067

第9节　癌前疾病　异型增生

原位癌................069

第10节　肿瘤发生的分子机制.......070

第11&12节　环境遗传致瘤因素

................071

Systemic pathology

073

Chapter 6   Diseases of Cardiovascular System 075

Section 1   Atherosclerosis 075

Section 2   Hypertension 080

Section 3   Rheumatism 085

Section 4   Subacute infective endocarditis 088

Section 5   Valvular heart disease 090

Section 6   Cardiomyopathy 093

Section 7   Myocarditis 095

Chapter 7   Diseases of Respiratory System 097

Section 1   Pneumonia 097

Section 2   Chronic obstructive pulmonary disease (COPD) 105

Section 3   Pneumoconiosis 113

Section 4   Tumors of respiratory system 114

Chapter 8   Diseases of Digestive System 117

Section 1   Gastritis 117

Section 2   Peptic ulcer 120

Section 3   Appendicitis 124

Section 4   Idiopathic inflammatory bowel disease (IBD) 126

病理学各论

073

第6章   心血管系统疾病 075

第1节   动脉粥样硬化 075

第2节   高血压 080

第3节   风湿病 085

第4节   亚急性感染性心内膜炎 088

第5节   心瓣膜病 090

第6节   心肌病 093

第7节   心肌炎 095

第7章   呼吸系统疾病 097

第1节   肺炎 097

第2节   慢性阻塞性肺疾病（COPD） 105

第3节   肺尘埃沉着症 113

第4节   呼吸系统肿瘤 114

第8章   消化系统疾病 117

第1节   胃炎 117

第2节   消化性溃疡 120

第3节   阑尾炎 124

第4节   炎症性肠病 126

Section 5 Viral hepatitis 130

Section 6 Cholecystitis and pancreatitis 134

Section 7 Liver cirrhosis 135

Section 8 Liver carcinoma 138

Section 9 Tumors of digestive tract 140

Chapter 9 Diseases of Lymphoid Tissue and Hematopoietic System 146

Section 1 Benign lesion of lymph node 146

Section 2 Lymphoid neoplasm: lymphoma 148

Chapter 10 Diseases of Urinary System 158

Section 1 Glomerular diseases 160

Section 2 Tubulointerstitial diseases 183

Section 3 Tumor of urinary system 186

Chapter 11 Diseases of Genital System and Breast 188

Section 1 Diseases of cervix 188

Section 2 Diseases of prostate........ 190

Section 3 Diseases of breast............ 191

第5节 病毒性肝炎......................... 130

第6节 胆囊炎和胰腺炎................. 134

第7节 肝硬化............................... 135

第8节 肝癌................................... 138

第9节 消化系统肿瘤..................... 140

第9章 淋巴造血系统疾病............ 146

第1节 淋巴结良性病变................. 146

第2节 淋巴组织肿瘤：淋巴瘤...... 148

第10章 泌尿系统疾病................. 158

第1节 肾小球疾病......................... 160

第2节 肾小管肾间质疾病............. 183

第3节 泌尿系统肿瘤..................... 186

第11章 生殖系统与乳腺疾病...... 188

第1节 宫颈疾病............................. 188

第2节 前列腺疾病......................... 190

第3节 乳腺疾病............................. 191

Chapter 12　Diseases of Endocrine System 194

Section 1　Diseases of the thyroid gland 194

Section 2　Diseases of the pancreatic islet 202

Chapter 13　Infectious Diseases 205

Section 1　Tuberculosis, TB 206

Section 2　Pulmonary tuberculosis 212

Section 3　Typhoid fever 218

Section 4　Bacillary dysentery 223

Section 5　Parasitosis 226

Section 6　Central nervous system disease 232

Section 7　Sexually transmitted disease (STD) 236

第 12 章　内分泌系统疾病 194

第 1 节　甲状腺疾病 194

第 2 节　胰岛疾病 202

第 13 章　感染性疾病（传染病）...... 205

第 1 节　结核病 206

第 2 节　肺结核 212

第 3 节　伤寒 218

第 4 节　细菌性痢疾 223

第 5 节　寄生虫病 226

第 6 节　中枢神经系统疾病 232

第 7 节　性传播疾病 236

Introduction to pathology
病理学绪论

Conception

- Pathology is a basic science devoted to understanding the causes of disease and the changes in cells, tissues, and organs that are associated with disease and give rise to the presenting signs and symptoms in patients
- Pathology is also a bridge between basic science and clinical medicine, which is concerned with the diagnosis and treatment of the diease entities

Classification

- Anatomical pathology is pathology, mainly concern the morphological changes of the disease and reveal the nature of the disease
- Pathophysiology is mainly discuss the functional changes of diseases during the development and progression of diseases

Status Quo

- Pathology provides the scientific basis for the medical practice
- "As is our pathology, so is our medicine." Sir William Osler said

Methodology（ABCDE）

- Autopsy also known as a post-mortem examination, is a special surgical

概述

- 病理学是研究疾病的原因、发病机制、病理变化、结局和转归的一门医学基础学科
- 病理学也是一座连接基础医学与临床医学的桥梁，主要关注疾病的诊断和治疗

分类

- **病理解剖学** 即病理学，主要观察疾病的形态变化，揭示疾病的本质
- **病理生理学** 主要研究疾病的功能改变，注重疾病的发生发展过程

现状

- 病理学为医学实践提供了科学依据
- "病理学为医学之本。"医学之父威廉·奥斯勒说

研究方法（ABCDE）

- **尸体剖验** 即尸检，是对死者的遗体和各器官进行检查以发现患者死

procedure to examine morphology of various organs on a dead body in order to identify the cause of death and correct diagnosis

- Biopsy   is the removal of a sample of tissue by forceps or special needle from the body for pathological examination and diagnosis of diseases
- Cytology   is responsible for preparation of diagnosis, which get patient samples or fluids for cytological smear by brushes needle aspiration
- Experimental pathology   is a reasearch to find out the pathological mechanism and assist in the diagnosis of diseases using animal models, cell culture and molecular biology methods

Development of pathology

- Organ pathology   was found by Morgagni in 18th century
- Cytopathology & Histopathology was found by Virchow in 19th century and Microscope was discovered
- Ultrastructual pathology   was found by the discovery electron microscope 20th century
- Molecular pathology   is introducing many biological methods to pathology in nowadays

亡的原因,并纠正诊断的方法

- **活体组织检查**   即活检,用局部切取、钳取、粗针穿刺和搔刮等手术方法从患者体内获取病变组织进行病理观察以明确疾病诊断的方法
- **细胞病理**   通过刷检、穿刺涂片或收集病变的液体或细胞涂片染色进行初步诊断的方法
- **实验病理**   运用动物模型,细胞培养和分子生物学方法等进行疾病研究,找出病理学规律,辅助疾病诊断的研究方法

病理学发展史

- **器官病理学**   18世纪 Morgagni 创立
- **细胞病理学和组织病理学**   19th Virchow 创立,光学显微镜诞生
- **超微结构病理**   20世纪 电子显微镜诞生
- **分子病理学**   现代病理学引入许多分子生物学方法

Pathology of Chinese medicine

- The Inner Canon of Huangdi
- General Treatise on the Cause and Symptoms of Disease
- Record of Redressing Mishandled Cases

Contents

General pathology

- Adaptation and Injury of Cells and Tissues
- Tissue Repair
- Disorders and Abnormalities of Local Blood Supply
- Inflammation
- Neoplasia

Systemic pathology

- Cardiovascular system
- Respiratory system
- Digestive system
- Urinary system
- Endocrine system
- Genital System and Breast
- Infectious diseases

How to study pathology

- We should connect the gross and histological examination and pay attention to pathological changes of diseases
- The pathological examination are including macroscopic, microscopic,

中医病理学

- 黄帝内经
- 诸病源候论

- 洗冤集录

内容

普通病理学

- 细胞和组织的适应与损伤

- 损伤的修复
- 局部血液循环障碍

- 炎症
- 肿瘤

系统病理学

- 心血管系统疾病
- 呼吸系统疾病
- 消化系统疾病
- 泌尿系统疾病
- 内分泌系统疾病
- 生殖系统与乳腺疾病
- 感染性疾病

如何学习病理学

- 我们应将宏观与微观相联系，重点观察疾病病理变化

- 病理检查包括肉眼、显微镜、超微结构、分子检测和临床特征

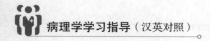

ultrastructural, molecular detection and clinical features

- The pathological characteristics of diseases are including general and special features
- Every disease should be concerned by etiology, pathogenesis, gross and microscopical features,clinical manifestations, outcomes and prognosis

- 疾病的病理特征包括基本病理特征和特殊病理特征

- 每一种疾病均应观察其病因、发病机制、肉眼与镜下特征、临床表现、结局以及预后

蒋　薇　何妙侠

General pathology

病理学总论

Chapter 1

Adaptation and Injury of Cell and Tissue

Section 1 Adaptation

Conception
Adaptation is the non-injury response of cells, tissues and organs to the stimulation of various harmful factors in the internal and external environment

Four Types of Adaptation
Atrophy
- Definition Atrophy is a decrease in the size of a cell, tissue and organ that have normally developed
- Causes Decreased of workload (e.g. immobilization of a limb to permit healing of a fracture), loss of innervation, diminished blood supply, inadequate nutrition, loss of endocrine stimulation and aging (senile atrophy)
- Classifications
  ○ Physical atrophy endometrium

第 1 章

细胞和组织的适应与损伤

第 1 节　适应

概述
适应　是细胞和由其构成的组织、器官对内外环境中各种有害因子的刺激作用而产生的非损伤性应答反应

四种适应类型
萎缩
- **定义**　已发育正常的细胞、组织或器官的体积缩小

- **原因**　萎缩的原因包括工作量下降（例如，固定肢体以使骨折愈合），神经支配力丧失，血液供应减少，营养不足，内分泌刺激丧失和衰老（老年性萎缩）

- **分类**
  ○ **生理性萎缩**　更年期后子宫内膜

atrophy after menopause

○ Pathological atrophy   Malnutritional atrophy; Compress atrophy; Unused atrophy; Denerved atrophy; Endocrinal atrophy; Ischemic atrophy

Hypertrophy

- Definition   Hypertrophy is referred to an increase in the size of cells, tissues or organs due to increased functions or synthetic metabolism
- Causes   Hypertrophy can be physiological or pathological, either from increased functional demands or from growth factor or hormonal stimulation
- Classifications
  ○ Physiological hypertrophy   e.g. uterus during pregnancy
  ○ Pathological hypertrophy   including compensatory pathological hypertrophy (e.g. cardiac enlargement) and endocrine pathological hypertrophy (e.g. tumors of endocrine organs)

Hyperplasia

- Definition   Hyperplasia is an increased number of parenchymal cells in a tissue or organ
- Classification
  ○ Different causes   Physiologic hyperplasia (compensatory, hormonal) and pathologic hyperplasia (excessive

萎缩

○ **病理性萎缩**   营养不良性；压迫性；失用性；去神经性；内分泌性；缺血性萎缩

肥大

- **定义**   由于功能增加、合成代谢旺盛，使细胞、组织或器官的体积增大
- **原因**   肥大可能是生理上或病理上的原因，既可能是功能需求增加，也可能是生长因子或激素刺激引起的
- **分类**
  ○ **生理性肥大**   例如怀孕期间的子宫
  ○ **病理性肥大**   包括代偿性病理性肥大（例如心脏扩大）和内分泌性病理性肥大（例如内分泌器官肿瘤）

增生

- **定义**   组织或器官内实质细胞的数目增多
- **分类**
  ○ **按原因分类**   生理性增生（代偿性，激素性）和病理性增生（过度激素或生长因子刺激）

hormonal or growth factor stimulation)

- Different patterns Diffuse hyperplasia (organ enlargement) and focally hyperplasia (nodular formation)

Metaplasia

- Definition Metaplasia is an abnormality of celluar differentiation in which one type of mature cell is replaced by another different type of mature cell

- Notes Metaplasia is not caused by the direct transformation of the original mature cells, but is the result of the transdifferentiation of stem cells or undifferentiated cells

- Classifications
  - Squamous metaplasia The most common type of epithelial metaplasia. Nonsquamous pseudo stratified columnar or cuboidal epithelium is replaced by stratified squamous epithelium
  - Intestinal metaplasia In chronic gastritis, the normal gastric mucosa epithelium may undergo metaplastic transformation to intestinal-type goblet cell
  - Mesenchymal metaplasia Osseous metaplasia occasionally in soft tissue
  - Epithelial-mesenchymal transformation A biological process in which epithelial cells are transformed

- 按程度分类 弥漫性增生(器官肿大)和局灶性增生(结节状形成)

化生

- 定义 一种分化成熟的细胞类型被另一种分化成熟的细胞类型所取代的过程

- 注意 化生并不是由原来的成熟细胞直接转变所致,而是该处具有分裂能力增殖和多向分化能力的干细胞或结缔组织中的未分化间充质细胞发生转分化的结果

- 分类
  - 鳞状上皮化生 最常见的上皮化生,非鳞状上皮的假复层柱状或立方上皮细胞被复层鳞状上皮细胞替代

  - 肠上皮化生 在慢性胃炎中,正常胃黏膜上皮发生转分化,转变为有杯状细胞的肠型上皮

  - 间质化生 在软组织中偶有骨化生
  - 上皮-间质转化 指上皮细胞通过转化为具有间质细胞表型的生物学过程

into mesenchymal phenotypes

Cellular Aging

- Definition Cellular aging is the result of a progressive decline in the life span and functional capacity of cells

Section 2 Causes and mechanism of cellular injury

Causes of cellular injury

- Hypoxia Oxygen supply reduced caused by respiratory disease, cardiovascular diseases and reducing blood supply. Loss of the oxygen-carrying capacity of the blood such as in anemia or carbon monoxide poisoning

- Physical factors such as mechanical trauma, extremely hot or cold temperatures, sudden change in atmospheric pressure, electrical shock and accident of irradiation

- Chemicals Any chemical or drug such as high glucose causes cell injury if sufficiently concentrated and derange the osmotic environment of the cell

- Microorganism A host of living organisms, ranging in size from the submicroscopic viruses to grossly

细胞老化

- 定义 细胞老化是细胞寿命和功能逐渐下降的结果

第2节 细胞损伤的原因和机制

细胞损伤的原因

- 缺氧 呼吸、心血管疾病以及血供下降均可导致氧气供应减少。血液携氧能力下降如贫血和一氧化碳中毒

- 物理因素 物理损伤如极端冷热、气压突然变化，电离辐射

- 化学制剂 任何化学物质或药物均可引起细胞损伤，如葡萄糖浓度太高导致细胞渗透压紊乱

- 微生物 任何生物，小至病毒大至线虫均可导致人类细胞损伤

visible nematodes, may attack human and cause cell injury

- **Abnormal immunological reactions** Hypersensitivity to various substances can lead to anaphylaxis or to more localized lesions. In other circumstances, the immune process may act against the body cells — autoimmunity

- **Genetic abnormality** Gene mutations may deprive the cell of a single enzyme. In some instances, the impacts are so severe that they could be incompatible with cell survival. Somatic mutations could lead to cancerous transformation of cells

- **Nutritional imbalances** Either lack of or excessive nutrition can damage cells. Excessive intake of calories and animal fat has been implicated in the development of atherosclerosis. Obesity alone leads to an increased vulnerability to certain disorders, such as atherosclerosis, coronary heart disease, diabetes mellitus

Mechanism of cellular injury

- Cell membrane injury
- Mitochondrial damage
- Damage by activated oxygen species
- Damage by calcium ions of cell
- Chemical damage

- **异常免疫反应** 对不同物质过于敏感可导致过敏症或局部病变。另外免疫反应对抗自身细胞可引起自身免疫

- **遗传异常** 基因突变导致酶异常,严重情况下引起细胞无法生存,体细胞突变易导致细胞恶性转化

- **营养失衡** 营养缺乏或过剩均可导致细胞损伤,摄入过多能量和动物脂肪与动脉粥样硬化发病有关。肥胖容易引起动脉粥样硬化、冠心病和糖尿病

细胞损伤机制

- 细胞膜损伤
- 线粒体损伤
- 活性氧类物质损伤
- 钙离子损伤
- 化学性损伤

- Genetic abnormality

- 遗传异常

Section 3　Reversible injury: Degeneration

第3节　可逆性损伤：变性

Definition

- Reversible injury also called degeneration
- Under some conditions, many normal and abnormal substances (endogenous or exogenous) maybe excessively accumulated either in the cytoplasm or in the interstitial tissues, always with decrease of cell function

定义

- 细胞可逆性损伤又叫变性
- 指细胞或细胞间质受损伤后，由于代谢障碍，细胞或细胞间质内出现异常物质或正常物质异常蓄积的现象，通常伴有细胞功能低下

Classification

- **Cellular swelling/hydropic degeneration**
  - **Definition**　Accumulation of fluid in the cytoplasm, which is the early slight injury of cells
  - **Causes**　Lack of oxygen; Toxic substance; Osmotic effect
  - **Mechanism**　Damaged mitochondria reduce ATP production, and the dysfunction of the cell membrane Na-K pump leads to excessive accumulation of intracellular Na^+ and water. Any damage that can cause changes in intracellular fluid and ion homeostasis will lead to this type of injury
  - **Grossly**　The size of the organ

分类

- **细胞水肿/水变性**
  - **定义**　细胞内水分聚集，是细胞损伤中最早最轻的改变
  - **病因**　缺氧；毒性物质；渗透效应
  - **机制**　线粒体受损，ATP减少，细胞膜Na-K泵的功能障碍导致细胞内钠离子和水过量蓄积。任何可能导致细胞内液和钠离子稳态变化的损伤都可能导致这种类型的损伤
  - **大体**　器官体积增大，包膜紧张，

is enlarged. Its fibrous capsule is tense. On the cut surface, the capsule is everted, and the color of the organ is pale and boiled-like

- ○ Morphologically   The cell volume is increased and its cytoplasm looks pale. it becomes and balloon-like with many fine particles

- Fatty change (Steatosis)
  - ○ Definition   Fatty change is the accumulation of triglyceride in the cytoplasm of non-fatty cells. The liver plays a central role in fatty metabolism and easily take fatty changes
  - ○ Grossly   Enlarged organs, blunt edges, grayish-yellow or yellowish, greasy on cut surface
  - ○ Morphologically   Lipid droplets or fat vacuoles can be seen in the cytoplasm
  - ○ Confirmation   Fat remains in the cytoplasm in frozen sections where it can be demonstrated by fat stains such as oil red O and Sudan Ⅲ (orange red)
  - ○ Tiger Heart   Fatty degeneration of the myocardium, often involving the subendometrial and papillary muscles of the left ventricle. The steatotic yellow myocardium has alternated with red normal one, called "tiger heart"

切面包膜外翻,色泽淡呈水煮样

- ○ 镜下   细胞体积增大,胞浆淡染,出现细颗粒状物,极期呈气球样

- 脂肪变
  - ○ 定义   甘油三酯蓄积于非脂肪细胞的细胞质中称为脂肪变。肝脏是脂肪代谢的重要场所,最常发生脂肪变性
  - ○ 大体   器官体积增大,边缘圆钝,淡黄色,切面有油腻感
  - ○ 镜下   细胞质内出现脂滴或脂肪空泡
  - ○ 确认   细胞质内脂肪在冰冻切片可以保留,并可以通过油红或苏丹Ⅲ脂肪染色证实
  - ○ 虎斑心   指心肌的脂肪变性,常累及左心室内膜下和乳头肌部位,脂肪变性的心肌呈黄色,与正常心肌的暗红色相间,形成黄红色斑纹,称为"虎斑心"

- Hyaline degeneration
  - Definition　It is applied to material of homogeneous, glassy, eosinophilic appearance accumulation in cytoplasm or interstitial on HE stained sections
  - Intracellular hyaline degeneration
    - Mallory bodies　are liver cell cytoplasmic aggregates of fragmented fine filaments
    - Russell bodies　are formed by immunoglobin in plasma cells
  - Collagenous fibrous tissue hyaline
    Scar tissue and atherosclerotic plaques
  - Arteriole wall hyaline degeneration
    High blood pressure causing hyaline degeneration of the arteriole wall
- Amyloid degeneration
  - Amyloid substance is composed essentially of an abnormal protein deposit in the extracellular tissue, particularly around blood vessels and basement membranes
- Mucoid degeneration
  - Mucoid degeneration is characterized by accumulation of mucin intracellular or extracellular matrix
- Pathological pigmentation
  - Pigments such as hemosiderin,

- 玻璃样变性
  - 定义　细胞胞内或间质中出现均质、玻璃样、嗜伊红物质蓄积, HE 染色呈嗜伊红均质状
  - 细胞内玻璃样变性
    - 马洛里小体　是肝细胞内聚集的中间丝蛋白
    - 拉塞尔小体　是浆细胞分泌的免疫球蛋白
  - 胶原纤维玻璃样变性

    多见于瘢痕组织, 动脉粥样硬化斑块
  - 细动脉壁玻璃样变性
    高血压引起的细小动脉壁玻璃样变
- 淀粉样变性
  - 由异常蛋白质组成的淀粉样物质沉积在细胞外组织中, 尤其是在血管和基底膜周围

- 黏液样变性
  - 以细胞内或细胞外基质中黏蛋白积聚为特征
- 病理性色素沉着
  - 含铁血黄素、脂褐素、黑色素、胆

lipofuscin, melanin, bilirubin, dust, pigment, etc. are accumulated inside and outside cells

- Pathologic calcification
  - Definition Abnormal deposits of calcium salts in any tissues except bones and teeth
  - Types Dystrophic calcification and metastatic calcification
  - Dystrophic calcification refers to the deposition of calcium salts in necrotic or foreign bodies, and the normal metabolism of calcium and phosphorus in the body, such as tuberculosis
  - Metastatic calcification refers to the deposition of calcium in normal tissues caused by systemic imbalance of calcium and phosphorus metabolism, such as hyperparathyroidism

Summary of Degeneration

- Intracellular Degeneration
  - Cellular swelling
  - fatty change
- Intracellular and extracellular
  - Hyaline degenration
  - Pathological pigmentation
  - Pathological calcification
- Extracellular Mucoid degenration
                      Amyloid degenration

红素、粉尘,色素等增多并积聚于细胞内外

- 病理性钙化
  - 定义 骨和牙齿之外的组织中固态钙盐沉积
  - 类型 营养不良性钙化和转移性钙化
  - 营养不良性钙化 指钙盐沉积在坏死或异物中,体内钙磷代谢正常,见于结核等
  - 转移性钙化 指由于全身钙磷代谢失调而致钙盐沉积于正常组织内,见于甲状旁腺功能亢进

变性小结

- 细胞内变性
  - 细胞水肿
  - 脂肪变
- 细胞内和细胞外变性
  - 玻璃样变性
  - 病理色素沉着
  - 病理性钙化
- 细胞外变性 黏液样变性
                  淀粉样变性

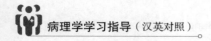

Section 4　Irreversible injury: Cell death

坏死 Necrosis

Definition

- Necrosis is a form of cell death characterized by enzymatically lytic changes in the living body

Basic pathologic changes

- Nuclear changes
  - Pyknosis is characterized by nuclear shrinkage and increased basophilia; the DNA condenses into a dark shrunken mass
  - Karyorrhexis is refers to the pyknotic nucleus become to fragmentation and dispersion in cytoplasm
  - Karyolysis is refers to digestion of DNA and nuclear proteins by deoxyribonuclease (DNase) activity, and nuclear chromatin becomes less basophilic and eventually disappear
- Cytoplasmic changes
  - Necrotic cells show increased eosinophilia
  - The cell may have a glassy, homogeneous appearance

第4节　不可逆性损伤：细胞死亡

坏死

定义

- 坏死　是以酶溶性变化为特点的活体内局部组织细胞的死亡

基本病理变化

- 细胞核变化
  - 核固缩　细胞核染色质DNA浓聚、皱缩，使细胞核体积减小、嗜碱性增强
  - 核碎裂　细胞核染色质崩解、发生碎裂，使核物质分散于胞质中
  - 核溶解　非特异性DNA酶和蛋白酶激活，分解核DNA核蛋白质，核染色质嗜碱性下降，最终消失

- 细胞质变化
  - 坏死细胞嗜酸性增强
  - 细胞呈均质玻璃样外观

Types of necrosis

- Coagulative necrosis
  - Defintion   Coagulative necrosis is a form of necrosis in which the underlying tissue architecture is preserved for at least several days after death of cells in the tissue
  - Cause   This type of necrosis is usually caused by the lack of blood supply and presumably the injury denatures not only structural proteins but also enzymes
  - Location   The affected tissues take on a firm texture. It is characteristic of infarcts in all solid organs such as liver except the brain
  - Grossly   Necrotic tissue shows gray-white area surrounded by hyperemia-bleeding zone demarcation from normal area
  - Microscopically   The necrotic cells show preserved outlines with loss of nuclei, and an inflammatory infiltrate is present
- Caseous necrosis
  - Definition   Caseous necrosis is a special coagulative necrosis often encountered in foci of tuberculous infection
  - Grossly   Caseous means "cheeselike", referring to the friable

坏死的类型

- 凝固性坏死
  - 定义   凝固性坏死是坏死组织的结构轮廓在坏死后保持若干天的一种坏死类型
  - 原因   局部缺乏血供,蛋白质变性凝固且溶酶体水解作用较弱
  - 部位   常见于脑以外的实质器官,如肝脏等
  - 大体   坏死组织灰白色、与周围与正常组织有充血—出血带分界
  - 镜下   细胞核消失,但组织结构轮廓存在

- 干酪样坏死
  - 定义   干酪样坏死是一种特殊类型的凝固性坏死,常发生于结核感染病灶中
  - 大体   干酪样像"奶酪样"指病灶坏死区易碎、色黄白的外观,是

yellow-white appearance of the area of necrosis. It is more complete coagulative necrosis

更彻底的凝固性坏死

○ Microscopically The necrotic focus appears as a collection of fragmented or lysed cells with an amorphous granular pink appearance in H&E stained tissue sections. The architecture is completely obliterated and cellular outlines cannot be discerned

○ 镜下 坏死灶溶解成碎片，H&E 切片上呈红染无结构的颗粒样物，组织结构和细胞轮廓均无法辨认

● Liquefactive necrosis

● 液化性坏死

○ Definition Liquefaction of necrotic cells results when lysosomal enzymes released by the necrotic cells cause rapid liquefaction

○ 定义 由于坏死细胞释放大量溶解酶而引起液化所致

○ Grossly The necrotic tissue looks like soft and liquid due to digesting and converting cells into a formless proteinaceous mass by enzymes released from neutrophils. Ultimately, the mass discharges its contents and forms a cystic space

○ 大体 病灶中看上去软、液状，坏死细胞被中性粒细胞等释放的溶解酶消化成无定型蛋白质团块，内容最终排出便形成空腔

○ Microscopically The necrotic cells are digested completely

○ 镜下 坏死细胞被完全消化

○ Fat necrosis is a special liquefactive necrosis in fat tissue, which usually forms grey calcium soap

○ 脂肪坏死 是一种特殊类型的液化性坏死，常发生于脂肪组织中，脂肪坏死后可形成灰白色钙皂

● Fibrinoid necrosis

● 纤维素样坏死

○ Definition Fibrinoid necrosis is immunologically mediated

○ 定义 是免疫反应介导的一种坏死，常发生于免疫性疾病和严重

reactions usually occur in immune diseases and severe hypertension

- ○ Location Connective tissue and small blood vessels
- ○ Microscopically Deposited immune complexes and plasma proteins that leak into the wall of damaged vessels produce a bright pink, amorphous appearance on H&E staining sections called fibrinoid (fibrinlike) by pathologists

- Gangrene
  - ○ Definition Gangrene is widely used in clinical situation in which extensive tissue necrosis is complicated to a variable degree by secondary bacterial infection
  - ○ Subtype Dry gangrene, Wet gangrene, gas gangrene
    - Dry gangrene most commonly occurs in the extremities as a result of ischemic necrosis of tissues due to arterial obstruction and the venous blood is normal. The necrotic area appears black, dry, and shriveled and is sharply demarcated from adjacent tissue. Secondary bacterial infection is usually in significant
    - Wet gangrene both arterial and venous obstruction. It occurs

的高血压

- ○ 部位 是结缔组织和小血管较常见的坏死形式
- ○ 镜下 血管壁出现免疫复合物或浆细胞蛋白沉积，H&E染色呈红染无定型样外观，病理学家称为纤维素样

- 坏疽
  - ○ 定义 局部组织大块坏死并继发细菌感染

  - ○ 类型 干性、湿性、气性坏疽

    - 干性坏疽 动脉阻塞而静脉回流通畅。多见四肢末端。坏死区干燥皱缩呈黑色。与正常组织分界明显，继发感染并不明显

    - 湿性坏疽 动脉阻塞且静脉回流受阻。多见于内脏或四肢。

in the extremities as well as in internal organs such as intestine. The necrotic area appears black, soft, swelling and is not demarcated from adjacent tissue. It results from severe bacterial infection superimposed on necrosis

- Gas gangrene a deep wound infection caused by *clostridium perfringens*. It is characterized by extensive necrosis of tissue and production of gas by fermentative action of the bacteria

Consequences of necrosis

- Digested by enzyme and phagocytosis by leukocyte
- Resolustion Isolated and Discharge by peripheral tissue formation of erosion; ulceration; sinus; fistula, cavity formation
  - Erosion is the superficial tissue defect of the skin or mucosa
  - Ulceration is a deep tissue defect of the skin or mucosa
  - Sinus is a deep ectopic duct opens only at the mucous surface or the skin
  - Fistula is a channel-like defect connecting two visceral organs or leading from visceral organs to the skin
  - Cavity is the remnant after

组织黑、软，肿胀，与正常组织分界不清。坏死基础上并发严重细菌感染

- **气性坏疽** 创伤伴产气荚膜杆菌感染。其特点是广泛坏死并发细菌发酵产生气体

坏死的结局
- 溶解和吸收

- **分离与排出** 坏死未被分离排出后形成糜烂、溃疡、窦道、瘘管和空腔

  - **糜烂** 皮肤、黏膜浅表组织缺损
  - **溃疡** 皮肤、黏膜较深的组织缺损
  - **窦道** 只开口于皮肤黏膜表面的深在性盲管
  - **瘘管** 连接两个内脏器官或从内脏器官通向体表皮肤的通道缺损
  - **空洞** 坏死物液化后经自然管道

liquefaction of necrotic material has been discharged through natural channels

- Organization and encapsulation Necrotic cells can be replaced with granulation tissue and collagen. Necrotic cells can be encapsulated by collagen called encapsulation
- Calcification   Necrotic area deposits by calcium salt and minerals called dystrophic calcification

Apoptosis

Definition

- Apoptosis has been used for individual cell death scattered in a population of healthy cells
- It differs from necrosis and represents a physiological process by which effete or abnormal cells die and are eliminated
- Also called programmed cell death

Mechanism

- Apoptosis is gene determined single cell death
- Apoptosis is important physiologically in balancing cell proliferation and elimination

Difference between necrosis and apoptosis

- Apoptosis   is a physiological process

排出后所残留的空腔

- 机化与包裹   新生肉芽组织长入并取代坏死组织、血栓、脓液、异物等过程称机化；如坏死组织等太大，则由周围的肉芽组织将其包围称为包裹

- 钙化   坏死组织未被及时清除，则吸引钙盐和矿物质沉积，称为营养不良性钙化

凋亡

定义

- 凋亡是活体内单个细胞散在性死亡

- 它不同于坏死，代表一种清除衰老或异常死亡的细胞的生理过程

- 亦称程序性细胞死亡

机制

- 凋亡是基因决定的单个细胞的死亡

- 凋亡在保存细胞增殖与消亡平衡上起着重要的作用

凋亡与坏死的区别

- 凋亡   是生理过程，由基因决定，凋

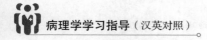
determined by genes. Apoptotic cells are scattered, forming apoptotic bodies, and DNA is regularly broken. It does not cause inflammation

- **Necrosis** is a pathological process caused by injury factors. Necrotic cells are distributed in sheets and their nuclei disappear. Necrosis often leads to inflammatory reactions

亡细胞散在，形成凋亡小体，DNA有规律断裂。不引起炎症反应

- **坏死** 是病理过程，由损伤因子所致，坏死细胞成片分布，细胞核消失，常引起炎症反应

蒋　薇　何妙侠

Chapter 2

Repair of injury

Conception

Repair is the process by which lost or destroyed cells are replaced by vital cells

Section 1 Repair by regeneration

Definition of Regeneration

The surviving healthy cells surrounding the damaged area proliferate and repair damaged tissue. Regeneration can also restore injured tissue to normal

Regeneration Types

- Complete regeneration Regenerated new tissue is the same as the lost one in both structure and function. It commonly occurs in physiological regeneration

第 2 章

损伤的修复

概述

修复是指损伤造成的机体部分细胞和组织丧失后,机体对所形成缺损进行修补恢复的过程

第 1 节 再生性修复

再生的定义

组织细胞损伤后,由周围同种细胞分裂增殖来完成修复的过程

再生的类型

- **完全性再生** 再生组织完全恢复原组织结构和功能,常见于生理状态的再生

○ The regenerative ability of parenchymal cells is strong

○ Damaged area is small and the stromal framework of the injured tissue is preserved well

- Incomplete regeneration Regenerative cells cannot restore the original tissue structure and function. The damaged tissue is repaired by granulation tissue and scars. It is commonly found in pathological regeneration

○ The regenerative ability of parenchymal tissue is weak

○ The damaged area is extensive and the stromal framework of the injured tissue is not preserved well

The potential regenerative ability of different types of cells

- Labile cells also known as continuously dividing cells. These cells are constantly proliferating to replace dying or destroyed cells, such as epidermal cells, respiratory and digestive tract mucosal lining cells hematopoietic cells, and mesothelial cells. More than 1.5% of the cells in the tissue are in the dividing stage. These tissue have stem cells

- Stable cells also known as quiescent cells. These cells are in the

○ 实质细胞再生能力很强

○ 损伤范围小，损伤组织的基质结构保存完好

- 不完全性再生 再生组织不能恢复原组织结构和功能，由肉芽组织修复，最后形成瘢痕。常见于病理性再生

○ 实质细胞再生能力较弱

○ 损伤范围广泛，损伤组织的基质结构破坏

不同细胞的再生能力

- 不稳定细胞 又称持续分裂细胞，这类细胞总在不断进行增殖，以代替衰老或破坏的细胞，如表皮细胞、呼吸和消化道黏膜被覆细胞、造血细胞、间皮细胞等。由其构成的组织超过1.5%的细胞处于分裂期。此类细胞存在干细胞

- 稳定细胞 又称静止细胞，处于G0期，损伤后进入G1期，如腺上皮、骨

G0 phase and enter the G1 phase after injury, such as glandular epithelium, osteoblasts, endothelial cells, smooth muscle cells, and parenchymal cells in liver, pancreas, kidney, etc. Less than 1.5% of the cells in the tissue are in the dividing stage. These tissue don't have stem cells

- Permanent cells   also called non-dividing cells. These cells are including neurons, myocardial cells and skeletal muscle cells. Normally, these cells have no capacity for mitotic division in postnatal life. Specially, peripheral nerve has retained the capacity for regeneration if neurons intact after damage

Stem cells

- Definition   Stem cell is a kind of cells with infinite or self-renewal and multidirectional differential ability in ontogenetic process
- Types
  - Embryonic stem cell
  - Adult stem cell
- Stem cell marker
  - CD34, CD133, c-Kit, CD44 etc.

Regeneration of different tissue

- Epithelial tissue
  - Injury to epithelial cells is followed by

母细胞、内皮细胞、平滑肌细胞,肝脏、胰腺和肾脏实质细胞等。由其构成的组织内处于分裂期的细胞少于1.5%。此类细胞不存在干细胞

- 永久细胞   又称非分裂细胞,包括如神经元、骨骼肌和心肌细胞等。通常情况下此类细胞在出生后都不能再分裂。而外周神经在神经细胞的存活下可以保存再生能力

干细胞

- 定义   干细胞是个体发育过程中产生的具有无限或较长时间自我更新和多向分化能力的一类细胞
- 类型
  - 胚胎干细胞
  - 成体干细胞
- 干细胞标记
  - CD34,CD133,c-Kit,CD44等

不同组织的再生

- 上皮组织
  - 黏膜的上皮损伤会快速再生,如

rapid regeneration, such as skin and digestive tract mucosa. The cells at the cut margins start to regeneration by division and migrate out as a thin layer over the denuded surface. Then the cells proliferation may result in a perfect restoration

○ If basement membrane is not destroyed, epithelial cells from the glands lining the basal layer can regenerate and restore glands to the origin structure. For example, if the liver plate framework is remain, the cells can restore complete, if not, may leads to disorder of liver cells arrangement and associate with liver cirrhosis

- Connective tissue
  ○ Fibrocytes   Located in loose connective tissues
  ○ Fibroblasts   Secretion of collagen including adhesive glycoproteins
  ○ Fibroblasts migration and proliferation in injury, then extracellular matrix deposit, at last, the fibrous tissue mature and reorganization.
- Blood vessels
  ○ Capillaries   Regeneration by sprout formation. The initial step in the growth of capillaries involves the enzymatic dissolution of the

皮肤和消化道黏膜。创缘或基底部残存的基底细胞分裂增生，向缺损中心覆盖

○ 腺上皮的损伤后，由残留的上皮细胞分裂、补充。例如，如果肝细胞板支架结构保持完好，细胞可以完全恢复，如果破坏，将会导致肝细胞排列紊乱，与肝硬化形成有关

- 结缔组织
  ○ 纤维细胞   存在于疏松结缔组织中
  ○ 成纤维细胞   分泌胶原纤维包括黏多糖
  ○ 损伤后成纤维细胞迁移和增生，然后细胞外基质沉积，最后纤维组织成熟和改建
- 血管
  ○ 毛细血管   再生以出芽方式完成，最初还包括毛细血管壁基底膜的酶溶性降解

basement membrane of existing capillaries

- ○ **Big blood vessels** Endothelial cells could be perfect restoration by complete regeneration; but smooth muscles of vessel wall are connected by scar

- **Muscle tissue**
  - ○ Smooth muscle cell can be restored in small vessels but not in big vessels
  - ○ Complete regeneration will done in large vessels, but smooth muscle cells should be connected by scar
  - ○ Regeneration of skeletal muscle cells are dependent on the intact of membrane of muscle bundle

- **Peripheral nerve**
  - ○ The basement membrane which surrounds the axon and Schwann cell remain intact, the peripheral nerve could be restored
  - ○ Axonal regeneration maybe accompanied by recovery of function of nerves

- **Bone and Cartilage**
  - ○ The periosteum on the surface of bone remains intact, the fractured bone could be regeneration after the correct orientation restored
  - ○ The injured cartilage is likely to be

- ○ **大血管** 内皮细胞完全再生，但是血管壁平滑肌则以瘢痕形式连接

- **肌肉组织**
  - ○ 小血管壁平滑肌可以恢复，但大血管壁不能

  - ○ 大血管的内皮细胞完全再生，但是血管壁平滑肌则以瘢痕形式连接
  - ○ 心肌和骨骼肌损伤后常形成瘢痕
  - ○ 骨骼肌的再生基于肌束周围肌膜是否完好无损

- **外周神经**
  - ○ 只要围绕在轴索周围的基底膜和鞘膜细胞完好无损，外周神经就能恢复

  - ○ 轴索的再生伴随神经功能的恢复

- **骨和软骨**
  - ○ 只要骨表面骨膜完好无损，骨折处在正确复位后就能再生

  - ○ 损伤的软骨通过纤维组织充填，

filled with fibrous tissues, or by the chondroblasts proliferate and transform to chondrocytes

或由软骨母细胞增生，转化为软骨细胞

Section 2　Repair by fibrinous tissue

第2节　纤维性修复

Granulation tissue

肉芽组织

Definition

定义

Granulation tissue is highly vascularized connective tissue composed of newly formed capillaries, proliferating fibroblasts, and residual inflammatory cells

由新生毛细血管、成纤维细胞及多少不等的炎症细胞构成

Morphology

形态

* Grossly　Granulation tissue is soft and fleshy and appearing pink, moist, and granular

* 肉眼　肉芽组织鲜红色、颗粒状、柔软湿润、似鲜嫩的肉芽

* Microscopically　There are fibroblasts; newly formed capillaries with thinner wall and big endothelial cells; inflammatory cells

* 镜下　包括成纤维细胞；新生的毛细血管，其内管壁薄，内皮细胞大；以及炎症细胞

Consequences

结局

* Granulation tissue is eventually replaced by scar tissue

* 肉芽组织最终被瘢痕组织替代

* Scar tissue is mainly composed of collagen fibers

* 瘢痕组织主要由胶原纤维构成

Functions

功能

* Filling wound or loss of tissue

* 填补缺损

* Anti-infection and protecting the surface of the wound

* 抗感染保护伤口

- Organization: granulation tissue replaces necrotic tissue, blood clot, and foreign bodies
- Encapsulation

Scar

- A scar is a mass of collagen that is the result of repair by organization and fibrosis
- Keloid is raised pinkish scar tissue at the site of an injury which results from excessive tissue repair
- Advantage of scar is to connect and fill wound
- Disadvantage of scar are including constriction, adhesion and keloid formation

Section 3　Healing of wound

Types of skin wound

Healing by the first intention

- Clean incised wounds with a minimum of space between the margins
- The wound edges are closely apposition

Healing by the second intention

- A wound will be left open and irregular
- Great tissue loss with more inflammatory exudates and necrotic material

- 机化：肉芽组织取代坏死组织、血凝块和异物
- 包裹

瘢痕

- 瘢痕是指修复后机化和改建形成的胶原团块
- 瘢痕疙瘩指损伤修复组织过度增生形成的突出于皮肤表面的粉色瘢痕组织
- 瘢痕有利的一面是可以连接和填补伤口
- 瘢痕不利的一面包括瘢痕收缩、粘连和瘢痕疙瘩形成

第3节　伤口愈合

皮肤伤口愈合类型

I期愈合

- 皮肤切口整齐,切缘空隙小
- 伤口对合整齐

II期愈合

- 皮肤伤口处缺口大且不规则
- 伤口处组织损失大,伴炎性渗出及坏死

- Increased liability to infection
- More granulation tissue, bigger scar and slower process

Healing of fractured bone

Stage of fractured bone healing

- **Hematoma** Initial connection
- **Provisional callus** Osteogenic granulation tissue, 3 days to 1 week

- **Bony callus** Osteoid tissue and bone tissue, 1 month
- **Bone remodeling** Osteoblast and osteoclast, several months

The factors influencing on fractured bone healing

- Timely and correct restoration of the fractured
- Timely and reliable fixations of broken
- Well blood supply of fractured bone
- Both exercises in local and whole body

- 容易感染
- 伤口修复需要更多肉芽组织、更多瘢痕，修复过程慢

骨折愈合

骨折愈合分期

- **血肿形成期** 初步连接
- **纤维性骨痂** 成骨性肉芽组织，3天至1周

- **骨性骨痂** 骨样组织及骨组织，1月

- **骨性骨痂改建** 成骨细胞、破骨细胞协同作用，改建需数月

骨折愈合的影响因素

- 骨折断端及时、正确复位

- 骨折断端及时、牢靠固定

- 局部良好的血液供应
- 全身和局部功能锻炼

何妙侠

Chapter 3
Local Blood Circulation Disorders

第3章
局部血液循环障碍

Section 1　Hyperemia and Congestion

第1节　充血和淤血

⚜ Conception

- Hemorrhage
  - A loss of blood from the vascular compartment during life
- Hyperemia and congestion
  - A local increased volume of blood in a particular tissue
- Hyperemia
  - Hyperemia is an active process
  - The blood flow is augmented after arteriolar dilation at local sites
  - Such as inflammation, exercise in skeleton muscle and stomach replete with food
  - The affected tissue is red and warm
- Congestion
  - Also called venous hyperemia resulting from impaired venous

⚜ 概念

- 出血
  - 血液从活体的血管或心腔溢出

- 充血和淤血
  - 局部血容量增加可引起充血和淤血
- 充血
  - 充血是主动过程
  - 局部组织由于小动脉扩展引起血流增加
  - 例如炎症、锻炼时的骨骼肌及充满食物的胃

  - 器官组织出现发热、发红
- 淤血
  - 淤血又称为静脉性充血,由静脉回流减少所致

return from a tissue
- ○ A passive process, such as cardiac failure or obstructive venous disease
- ○ The tissue is cool, edema, and blue-gray in color called cyanosis

Venous congestion in heart failure

- ● Pulmonary venous congestion
  - ○ Left heart failure causes congestion of the pulmonary circulation
  - ○ Acute pulmonary congestion
    - ● Grossly The lung weight is increased; the cut surface of lung is full of frothy hemorrhagic fluid
    - ● Microscopically Dilation of alveolar capillaries with transudation of fluid into the alveoli which full of red cells and pink exudation
  - ○ Chronic pulmonary congestion
    - ● The long-standing increase in pulmonary venous pressure stimulates development of fibrosis in alveolar walls
    - ● Grossly The lung hard, stenosis with brown in color called Brown induration of the lung
    - ● Microscopically The alveoli septa become thickened and

- ○ 淤血是被动过程，见于心力衰竭和静脉回流受阻
- ○ 器官组织凉，水肿，呈蓝灰色，又称为发绀

心衰性静脉淤血

- ● 肺淤血
  - ○ 左心衰竭 引起的肺循环淤血

  - ○ 急性肺淤血
    - ● 大体 肺重量增加，切面充满出血性泡沫状液体

    - ● 镜下 肺泡壁毛细血管扩张，肺泡腔水肿，充满红细胞和粉红色水肿液

  - ○ 慢性肺淤血
    - ● 长期肺静脉受压导致肺泡壁纤维组织增生

    - ● 大体 肺质地变硬、纤维化，呈棕褐色，称为肺褐色硬化

    - ● 镜下 慢性肺淤血使肺泡壁增厚纤维化，巨噬细胞吞噬大量

fibrosis, macrophages phagocytose red cell in the alveoli then the red cell was broken down into hemosiderin granules called heart failure cells

- Hepatic venous congestion
  - Right heart failure causes congestion of systemic circulation
  - The pressure of the right heart chamber increases, the hepatic venous return is blocked, and the blood accumulates in the hepatic lobular veins, resulting in the expansion and congestion of the central hepatic veins and hepatic sinusoids
  - Acute hepatic congestion
    - Grossly   The volume of liver becomes larger with dark red in color
    - Microscopically   Dilation of the central hepatic veins and congestion of the sinusoids
  - Chronic hepatic congestion
    - Grossly   The central regions of hepatic lobules are red-brown and slightly depressed while the peripheral zones are tan and pale sometimes fatty, then create a mottled effect called Nutmeg liver
    - Microscopically   There is

红细胞,形成含有大量含铁血黄素的巨噬细胞称为**心衰细胞**

- 肝淤血
  - 右心衰竭所致的全身循环障碍

  - 右心腔压力升高,肝静脉回流受阻,血液淤积在肝小叶静脉内,致使肝小叶中央静脉及肝窦扩张淤血

  - 急性肝淤血
    - **大体**   肝脏体积增大,呈暗红色

    - **镜下**   肝小叶中央静脉扩张及肝窦淤血

  - 慢性肝淤血
    - **大体**   肝中央静脉中心区域红棕色,而肝小叶周边区呈淡白色,有时似脂肪样,构成红黄相间的槟榔样称为**槟榔肝**

    - **镜下**   肝小叶中央区肝细胞坏

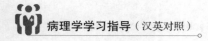

evidence of centrilobular necrosis with hepatocyte drop-out and hemorrhage, including hemosiderin-laden macrophages, while peripheral zones are fatty changes because of congestion

- **Congestive liver cirrhosis** Also called cardiac cirrhosis. The cells in the central zone of the liver lobule may eventually undergo necrosis and then fibrosis while the survival peripheral zonal cells may result in a nodular liver

死、消失伴出血,肝小叶周边部肝细胞因淤血而脂肪变性

- **淤血性肝硬化** 又称为心源性肝硬化,肝小叶中央区域肝细胞坏死最终伴纤维化,而周边部残存肝细胞呈结节状

Section 2　Thrombosis

Conception

- The formation of a blood clot within the vascular system in the body called thrombosis
- The blood clot is called thrombus

The condition of thrombosis

- Cardiovascular endothelial injury
  - Endothelium damage is the dominant influence and lead to thrombosis
  - Injury to the vascular endothelium leading to subendothelial collagen

第2节　血栓形成

概述

- 在活体的心脏和血管内,血液发生凝固或血液中某些有形成分凝集形成固体质块的过程称为**血栓形成**
- 所形成的固体称为**血栓**

血栓形成的条件

- 心血管内皮细胞的损伤
  - 内皮细胞损伤是血栓形成的最主要因素
  - 血管内皮损伤后暴露内皮下胶原具有很强的血栓生成效应,促其

exposure has a strong thrombogenic effect on platelets and results in the adherence of collagen

与胶原黏附

- The intrinsic pathway, initiated activation of Factor XII; The extrinsic coagulation pathway, initiated by tissue factor

- 激活血小板和凝血因子XII，启动了内源性凝血过程；同时损伤的内皮细胞释放组织因子，激活凝血因子VII，启动外源性凝血过程

- Thrombosis derived from the platelets adhering to the injured endothelium platelets at the site

- 血栓形成始于受损伤的血管内皮

- Such as hypertension, injured valves, bacterial endocarditis, and operation

- 例如高血压、瓣膜受损、细菌性心内膜炎和手术等

- Alterations in normal blood flow
  - Normal blood flow is laminal such that platelet elements flow centrally in the vessel lumen, separated from the endothelium by a slower moving clear zone of plasma

- 血流状态改变
  - 正常血流是分层的，血小板等位于血管中间的轴流与位于边流的血浆分开，不易接触到血管内皮

  - Stasis is a major factor in the development of venous thrombi

  - 血液淤滞是静脉血栓形成的主要因素

  - Stasis and turbulence disrupt laminal flow and bring platelets into contact with the endothelium

  - 血液淤滞或湍流打破了血液层流，导致血小板容易接触血管内皮

  - Such as atherosclerotic plaque, mitral valve stenosis, aneurysm and stay in bed for a long time

  - 例如动脉粥样硬化斑块、二尖瓣狭窄、动脉瘤、长期卧床等

- Hypercoagulability
  - Any alteration of the coagulation pathways that predisposes to the thrombosis

- 血液凝固性增加
  - 任何原因导致血液凝固性改变均易导致血栓形成

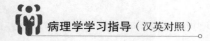
- It can be divided into primary and secondary disorders, the former one is the inherited hypercoagulability
- Secondary following surgery or trauma; in pregnancy and parturition; in some users of the oral contraceptive pill; after splenectomy; in endotoxic shock, hypersensitivity reactions; with some tumors

Types of thrombi

- Pale thrombus
  - The pale thrombus is the thrombus often in the fast-flowing arterial circulation such as coronary, cerebral, and femoral arterials, it is also at the head of venous thrombus
  - The pale thrombi are composed of fibrin and platelets
  - The pale thrombi are firmly adherent to the injured arterial wall and gray-white and friable
- Red thrombus
  - The red thrombi typically occur in venous system, where the slower blood flow encourages trapped red cells. It is at the end part of venous thrombus
  - The red thrombi are composed of platelets, fibrin and large number of erythrocytes trapped in the fibrin

- 可以分为原发性和继发性，原发性常常为遗传性高凝血症
- 继发性见于大手术或创伤后，怀孕和分娩时，某些口服避孕药的使用者，脾切除后，内毒素休克，超敏反应和某些肿瘤

血栓类型

- 白色血栓
  - 白色血栓常位于血流较快的动脉循环如冠状动脉，脑动脉和四肢动脉，也位于静脉血栓的头部
  - 白色血栓由血小板及纤维蛋白构成
  - 白色血栓呈灰白色，很牢固地黏附于受损的动脉壁
- 红色血栓
  - 红色血栓发生在静脉系统，血流较慢，卷入大量红细胞，常见于静脉血栓的尾部
  - 红色血栓由血小板、纤维蛋白及纤维蛋白网住的大量红细胞构成

mesh

- Mixed thrombus
  - Mixed thrombus often arises in the slowly moving venous blood forming body of venous thrombus
  - The blood flow moves slowly after original part of pale thrombus, and then number of erythrocytes coagulate
  - Mixed thrombi contain the pale layers of platelets and fibrin that alternate with dark-red layers containing more red cells
- Hyaline thrombus or microthrombus
  - Microthrombus usually appears in DIC
  - Numerous microthrombus are seen in microcirculation in capillaries
  - Microthrombus is composed of fibrin

Outcomes of thrombosis

- Fibrinolysis
  - Lysis of thrombus accompanied by reestablished of the lumen is the ideal result
- Organization and Recanalization
  - Thrombus organization The gradual replacement of blood clots by granulation tissue
  - Thrombus recanalization During the process of thrombus organization,

- 混合血栓
  - 混合血栓常见于血流较慢的静脉,是构成静脉血栓的主干
  - 缓慢的血流起始于白色血栓,然后是大量红细胞的凝固
  - 混合血栓包含血小板和纤维蛋白构成的白色层和红细胞构成的暗红色层形成红白相间的结构
- 透明血栓(微血栓)
  - 微血栓最常见于血管内弥散性凝血(DIC)
  - 微循环的毛细血管内可见大量微血栓
  - 微血栓由纤维蛋白构成

血栓的结局

- 溶解吸收
  - 血栓溶解吸收后恢复正常血流是最好的结局
- 机化和再通
  - **血栓机化** 由肉芽组织逐渐取代血栓的过程
  - **血栓再通** 在血栓机化过程中形成新的通道使血流重建

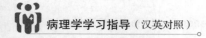

new channels across through thrombus and maybe some blood flow restored

- ○ Organization and recanalization commonly occur in large thrombi
- Calcification
  - ○ The longstanding thrombus usually secondary shows calcification
  - ○ Venous thrombus calcification also called phlebolith

- ○ 机化和再通　常见于大的血栓

- 钙化
  - ○ 血栓长时间存在可继发钙化

  - ○ 静脉血栓钙化称为静脉石

Section 3　Embolism

Conception

- **Embolism** is the occlusion or obstruction of a vessel by an abnormal mass (solid, liquid, or gaseous) transported from a different site by the circulation
- **Emboli** Most emboli are detached fragments of thrombi that carried in the bloodstream to the original site

Pathway of emboli

- Origin in systemic vein
  - ○ Emboli from right side of the heart system or venous system lodge in the pulmonary arterial system unless they are so small
  - ○ The point of lodgment in the

第3节　栓塞

概念

- **栓塞**　在循环血液中出现的不溶于血液的异常物质，随血液运行阻塞血管腔的现象

- **栓子**　阻塞血管腔的异常物质

栓子的运行途径

- 静脉系统及右心血栓
  - ○ 来自静脉系统及右心血栓引起肺动脉及其分支栓塞

  - ○ 肺动脉栓塞的关键是血栓的大小

pulmonary arterial circulation depends on the size of embolus

- Origin in heart and systemic arteries
  - Emboli from left side of the heart and systemic or arteries lodge in the distal arterial system such as brain, spleen, kidney, extremity
- Portal venous systemic emboli
  - Emboli that originate in branch of the portal vein lodge in the liver such as cancer cells from pancreas
- Paradoxical embolism
  - An embolus originating in a systemic vein passes across a defect in the cardiac interatrial or interventricular septum to lodge in systemic artery
- Retrograde embolism
  - An embolus in the inferior venous system, due to a sudden increase in chest cavity or abdominal pressure, temporarily refluxes the embolus to the branches of the liver, kidneys, or iliac veins

Types of Embolism

- Thromboembolism
  - Detached fragments of a thrombi are the most common cause of thromboembolism
- Pulmonary embolism
  - More than 95% embolus are from

- 主动脉系统及左心血栓
  - 来自动脉系统或左心的血栓阻塞各器官小动脉,常见于脑、脾、肾及四肢

- 门静脉系统栓子
  - 引起肝内门静脉分支的栓塞,如胰腺癌栓子

- 交叉性栓塞
  - 来自右心或腔静脉系统的血栓,在右心压力升高的情况下通过先天性房(室)间隔缺损到达左心,再进入体循环系统引起栓塞
- 逆行性栓塞
  - 下腔静脉内血栓由于胸腹压突然升高,使血栓一时性逆流至肝、肾、髂静脉分支并引起栓塞

栓塞类型

- 血栓栓塞
  - 由血栓脱落引起的栓塞是最常见的血栓性栓塞

- 肺动脉栓塞
  - 95%以上栓子来自于下肢及深部

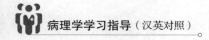

lower limb and deep venous, especially from popliteal vein, femoral vein, iliac vein

静脉如腘静脉、股静脉、髂静脉

○ Large embolus lodges at large branch of pulmonary arteries, small-medium emboli to small pulmonary arteries, numerous small emboli block pulmonary small arteries

○ 大栓子常形成肺动脉栓塞；中小栓子常堵塞肺小动脉；多量小栓子常导致较多肺小动脉分支栓塞

○ Massive emboli could cause sudden death probably because of severe vasoconstriction and smooth muscle constriction of bronchi, and acute right heart failure

○ 大栓子常致猝死，其原因包括动脉和支气管平滑肌痉挛和急性右心衰竭

- Systemic arterial embolism
  - ○ The detached thrombus originates in the left side of the heart or a large artery led to thromboembolism

- 体循环动脉栓塞
  - ○ 来自于左心或大动脉的栓子常导致血栓性栓塞

  - ○ Infarction is common when emboli lodge in the arteries of different organs such as brain, kidney, and spleen

  - ○ 常常引起不同器官如脑、肾、脾的梗死

- Fat embolism
  - ○ Fat embolism occurs when globules of fat enter the bloodstream

- 脂肪栓塞
  - ○ 脂肪损伤见于循环血流中出现脂肪滴阻塞小血管

  - ○ It is typically after fractures of large bones have exposed the fatty bone marrow

  - ○ 常见于长骨骨折时暴露骨髓中的脂肪

  - ○ Circulating fat globules first encounter the capillary network of the lung

  - ○ 循环脂滴常常首先堵塞肺毛细血管

- Air embolism
  - ○ Air embolism occurs when enough

- 空气栓塞
  - ○ 空气栓塞发生于大量空气迅速进

air bubbles enter the vascular system produce clinical symptoms

- Air embolism occurs in the situation of surgery, childbirth, and trauma
- **Decompress sickness** is a form of embolism occurs in caisson workers and under-sea drivers if they ascend rapidly after submerged for a long period. When air is breathed under high underwater pressure, an increased volume of air, mainly oxygen and nitrogen, goes into solution in the blood and equilibrates in the tissues. If decompressed to sea level too rapid, the gases that have equilibrates in the tissues come out of solution

- Amniotic fluid embolism
  - The contents of the amniotic fluid may rarely enter rupture uterine venous sinus during labor in childbirth
  - Amniotic fluid is rich in thromboplastic substances such as fetal squamous epithelium, fetal hair, fat and mucin, that induce disseminated intravascular coagulation (DIC)
- Tumor embolism
  - Cancer cells often enter the circulation during metastasis of malignant tumors

入血循环引起临床症状

- 多见于外科手术、分娩和创伤时

- **减压病** 是指沉箱工人或深海工作者潜水长时间后上升太快所致。人在水下高压下吸入空气时，大量的空气（主要是氧和氮）会在血液中溶解，并在组织中达到平衡，如果减压到海平面的速度过快，在组织中达到平衡的气体就会从溶液中释放出来导致减压病

- **羊水栓塞**
  - 分娩时羊水内容物很少进入破裂的子宫静脉窦内
  - 羊水内容物富有促血栓形成的物质如胎儿皮脂、毛发、脂肪和黏液等常引起弥散性血管内凝血（DIC）

- **肿瘤栓塞**
  - 恶性肿瘤转移时癌细胞常常进入血流循环

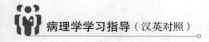

○ Large fragment of cancer cells may lead to emboli such as renal carcinoma and hepatic carcinoma

○ 癌细胞形成大的碎片可以导致栓塞，如肾癌和肝癌

Section 4 Infarction

第4节 梗死

Conception

- Infarction is an area of ischemic necrosis within a tissue or an organ resulting from decrease of blood supply
- Both of parenchymal cells and interstitial tissue undergo necrosis
- Infarction is most commonly due to arterial obstruction

概念

- 器官或局部组织由于血管阻塞、血流停止导致缺氧而发生的坏死

- 梗死局部实质和间质均可发生坏死

- 常由动脉阻断而引起

Types of infarctions

- Anemic infarct
  ○ Also called white infarct
  ○ Anemic infarcts occur because of arterial obstruction in solid organ such as spleen, kidney, heart, and brain
  ○ The artery branch is blocked, the local tissue is ischemic and hypoxic without enough collateral supply
  ○ The infarcts are grayish white in cut surface, infarcts in spleen and kidney are wedge-shaped like cone. Brain and myocardial infarctions are irregular in shape determined by the

梗死类型

- 贫血性梗死
  ○ 又称为白色梗死
  ○ 发生于实质器官动脉阻断，如脾、肾、心肌和脑组织

  ○ 当动脉阻断时局部缺血缺氧，侧支循环不丰富时

  ○ 梗死灶切面灰白色，发生于脾、肾的梗死灶呈锥形，脑和心肌则呈不规则地图状

distribution of the occluded artery

○ The margin between the infarct and normal tissue is clear with hyperemic and hemorrhagic band due to inflammation

- Hemorrhagic infarct
  ○ Also called red infarct
  ○ Hemorrhagic infarcts occur in tissues that have double blood supply such as lung and liver, or intestine that have collateral vessels permitting some continued flow into the area
  ○ It is associated with severe congestion loose tissues
  ○ Lung hemorrhagic infarction always located the lower lobe as cone in shape, the apex of infarct is to hilum of lung
  ○ Intestinal infarction mostly common occur in the small intestine because of occlusion of the superior mesentery artery and develop in loops of bowel in accordance with the pattern of arterial supply
- Septic infarct
  ○ Septic infarcts occur in situations where there is an infarction with additional infection such as acute infective endocarditis

○ 梗死灶与正常组织界限清楚,可见因炎症反应出现充血出血带

- 出血性梗死
  ○ 又称为红色梗死
  ○ 常见于双重供血的器官,动脉阻塞同时伴有静脉阻塞如肺和肝,肠梗死则于侧支循环不断由血液流入所致
  ○ 发生条件严重淤血、组织疏松
  ○ 肺出血性梗死多位于肺下叶,呈锥形或楔形,尖部指向肺门
  ○ 肠出血性梗死多发生于小肠是因为肠系膜上动脉阻塞,形状呈环状是因为血管分布的特点

- 败血性梗死
  ○ 由含有细菌的栓子阻塞血管引起,常见于急性感染性心内膜炎

顾昊煜　何妙侠

Section 1   Conception of inflammation

Conception

- Inflammation is a complex reaction to injurious agents that consists of vascular response, cellular and systemic reactions
- Inflammation is a delicately integrated defensive process
- Inflammation is divided into acute and chronic inflammation based on the process and duration

Basic pathological changes

- Alteration   refers degeneration and necrosis of local tissues and cells in inflammatory response
- Exudation   The process of fluid and cellular components in the blood vessels exudate out to interstitial tissues, body cavities or mucosal

第 1 节   炎症概述

概述

- 炎症是具有血管系统的活体组织对损伤因子所发生的复杂防御反应

- 炎症是精细的防御过程

- 炎症根据发病过程和持续时间分为急性和慢性炎症

基本病理变化

- 变质   炎症局部组织、细胞发生的变性和坏死

- 渗出   炎症局部组织血管内的液体和细胞成分通过血管壁进入组织、体腔、体表和黏膜表面的过程

surfaces through the vessel wall

- Hyperplasia Both of parenchyma and interstitial cells proliferate

Clinical Manifestations

- Local signs
  - Redness (Rubor)
  - Swelling (Tumor)
  - Increased heat (Calor)
  - Pain (Dolor)
  - Dysfunction (Functio laesa)
- System Symptoms
  - Fever
  - Neutrophil leukocytosis Increased of white blood cell counts

Significance

- Advantage
  - Dilutes, neutralizes, kills, and surrounds injury factors
  - Repairing and healing injured tissues through regeneration of parenchymal and stromal cells
- Disadvantage
  - Excessive exudate may cause dysfunction of related organs
  - The inflammatory response can also cause dysfunction of organ

Classification

- Acute inflammation Alteration and

- 增生 实质细胞和间质细胞的增生

临床表现

- 局部
  - 红
  - 肿
  - 热
  - 痛
  - 功能障碍
- 全身
  - 发热
  - 外周血白细胞增高

意义

- 有利
  - 稀释、中和、杀伤和包围损伤因子
  - 同时通过实质和间质细胞的再生使受损伤的组织得以修复和愈合
- 不利
  - 渗出液过多时可造成相关器官的功能障碍
  - 炎症的修复反应也能引起机体功能障碍

分类

- 急性炎症 变性和渗出

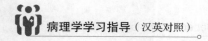

exudation
- Chronic inflammation Hyperplasia

- 慢性炎症 增生

Section 2   Acute inflammation

第2节   急性炎症

Conception

- Acute inflammation is rapid response to inflammatory agents in the early stage
- Exudation of fluid and emigration of leukocytes from blood vessels to the area of injury
- Acute inflammation lasts less than 1 month

概述

- 急性炎症是对致炎因子早期的快速反应
- 以变质和渗出性病变为主

- 持续时间短，<1个月

Vascular reaction

- Microcirculatory Response
  ○ Vasodilation transient and insignificant vasoconstriction
  ○ Then followed by marked active dilation of arterioles, capillaries, and venules
  ○ Then blood flow becoming slow as stasis
- Increased Permeability (fluid exudate)
  ○ Endothelial cell contraction increased the separation of intercellular functions from one to another
  ○ Transport activities was enhanced through the endothelial barrier

血管反应

- 血流动力改变
  ○ 细动脉短暂收缩
  ○ 血管扩张和血流加速
  ○ 血流速度减慢
- 血管通透性增加（液体渗出）
  ○ 内皮细胞收缩，内皮间缝隙增大
  ○ 内皮细胞穿胞作用增强

- Direct damaged of vascular endothelial cells
- High permeability of new blood vessels
- High permeability of vessels leads to exudate of fluid
- The difference between exudate and transudate is mainly permeability of vessels

Leukocytic response

- Exudation of Leukocytes
  - Leukocyte margination   Leukocytes in the capillary and small veins leave the center of the blood vessel (axial flow) to the periphery of the blood vessel (lateral flow) because of slow blood flow and fluid exudation
  - Leukocyte rolling   Leukocytes run over the surface of endothelial cells and then adhere to them at times
  - Leukocyte adhesion   Leukocytes adhere firmly to the surface of endothelial cells
  - Leukocyte emigration   The leukocytes leave post capillary venule through intercellular junction. Neutrophils swam out first in the early stage, and monocytes are dominated after neutrophils
  - Chemotaxis   The leukocytes

- 血管内皮细胞损伤
- 新生毛细血管的高通透性
- 血管通透性增加导致液体渗出
- 渗出液和漏出液区别的关键点是血管壁通透性

白细胞反应

- 白细胞渗出
  - 白细胞边集   随着血流缓慢和液体渗出的发生，毛细血管后静脉中的白细胞离开血管的中心部（轴流），到达血管的周边部（边流）
  - 白细胞滚动   白细胞在内皮细胞表面翻滚，并不时黏附于内皮细胞
  - 白细胞黏附   白细胞牢固地黏附于内皮细胞的表面
  - 白细胞游出   血管内白细胞逸出血管进入周围组织的过程
  - 趋化作用   白细胞沿化学物质浓

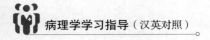

move to the direction along the chemical gradient toward the site of injury. Chemotactic factors are the chemicals that govern the movement of leukocytes

- Activation of leukocytes
  - Activation of leukocytes may be caused by pathogens, necrotic debris, antigen-antibody complexes, and cytokines
  - Opsonin is a group of proteins that enhance the capability of phagocytos is enveloping microorganisms and help macrophage of recognition
  - Opsonization is the process through coating agents such as antibody IgG or complement C3b encases microorganisms to enhance phagocytosis
  - Phagocytosis is the neutrophil and macrophage recognized organisms through the receptors on the surface and then attachment, engulfment, killing and degradation
- Features of leukocytes
  - Neutrophils emigrate in the early stage of inflammation, acute inflammation, purulent inflammation
  - Macrophages emigrate in the late stage of inflammation, chronic inflammation, non-purulent inflammation

度梯度向着化学刺激物做定向移动。**趋化因子**是指具有吸引白细胞定向移动的化学刺激物

- 白细胞的激活
  - 可由病原体、坏死细胞碎屑、抗原抗体复合物和细胞因子引起

  - **调理素** 是一类通过包裹微生物而增强吞噬细胞吞噬功能的血清蛋白质

  - **调理素化** 是指抗体IgG或补体C3b包裹微生物提高吞噬细胞吞噬作用的过程

  - **吞噬作用** 是指中性粒细胞和巨噬细胞通过表面的受体附着、吞入、杀灭和降解微生物

- 白细胞的特征
  - **中性粒细胞** 常出现于炎症早期、急性炎症和化脓性炎症

  - **巨噬细胞** 常见于炎症晚期、慢性炎症和非化脓性炎症

○ Plasma cells emigrate in the immune reaction and eosinophils infiltrate in parasite and allergic inflammation

Inflammatory mediators

- Definition Inflammatory mediators are a variety of endogenic chemical substances play some important roles in the modulation of inflammatory response
- The role of inflammatory mediators is vascular dilation, permeability increasing and leucocyte exudation
- Components
  ○ Cell-derived mediators
    - Vasoactive amines Histamine, Serotonin (5–HT)
    - Arachidonic acid (AA) metabolic products prostaglandins (PG), Leukotriene (LT), and lipoxins(LX)
    - Platelet activating factor (PAF)
    - Cytokine TNF and IL-1
  ○ Plasma-derived mediators
    - Kinin system Bradykinin
    - Complement system C3a C3b C5a C5b
    - Clotting system Thrombin

Types of acute inflammation

- Serous inflammation
  ○ Mainly exudate with serous, watery,

○ 浆细胞常见于免疫反应, 嗜酸性粒细胞常见于寄生虫感染及过敏性炎症

炎症介质

- 定义 参与并介导炎症反应的化学因子
- 作用 血管扩张、通透性增加和白细胞渗出
- 主要成分
  ○ 细胞释放的炎症介质
    - 血管活性胺 组胺、5-羟色胺
    - 花生四烯酸代谢产物 前列腺素、白细胞三烯、脂质素
    - 血小板激活因子
    - 细胞因子 TNF 和 IL-1
  ○ 体液中的炎症介质
    - 激肽系统 缓激肽
    - 补体系统 C3a、C3b、C5a、C5b
    - 凝血系统 凝血酶

急性炎症类型

- 浆液性炎症
  ○ 以浆液渗出为主要特征, 渗出物

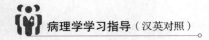

low protein content, derived from blood or serosal lining cells

○ It was commonly seen in mucosa, skin, peritoneal, pleural, and pericardial cavities

○ Catarrhal inflammation is inflammation on the surface mucosa with serous hypersecretion

- Fibrinous inflammation

  ○ Severe injuries cause greater increasing in vascular permeability

  ○ Large amounts of fibrinogen pass the vessel wall and form fibrins forming pseudo-membrane

  ○ It was commonly seen in serosa, lung, mucous membrane, such as throat (diphtheriae), cardiac cavity (Cor villosum) and intestine (bacillary dysentery)

  ○ When fibrinous inflammation of the mucosa forming a pale membrane covering the mucosal surface with exudate fibrin, necrotic substance, and inflammatory cells called pseudomembrane

- Suppurative/purulent inflammation

  ○ It is characterized by the formation of purulent exudates or pus

  ○ Pus is made of neutrophils, necrotic cells and fluid, and pyogenic organisms

以血浆成分为主

○ 常发生于黏膜、皮肤、腹膜、胸腔和心包腔等

○ 卡他性炎是指发生于黏膜表面的以浆液分泌为主

- 纤维素性炎症
  ○ 严重损伤导致血管通透性增加

  ○ 以纤维蛋白原渗出为主，继而在病灶中形成纤维蛋白假膜

  ○ 易发生于黏膜、浆膜和肺组织如喉部（白喉）、心包腔（绒毛心）和肠黏膜（菌痢）

  ○ 黏膜的纤维素性炎，渗出的纤维素、坏死组织和炎细胞共同形成一层覆盖于黏膜表面的灰白色膜状物称为**假膜**

- 化脓性炎症
  ○ 以中性粒细胞渗出为主，并有不同程度的组织坏死和脓液形成为特征的炎症
  ○ 多由化脓菌感染所致，亦可由组织坏死继发感染所致脓性渗出物

称为脓液, 脓液中的中性粒细胞大多数已发生变性和坏死, 称为脓细胞

- Surface purulent inflammation is purulent inflammation of mucosal or serosa surface

- 表面化脓是发生在黏膜和浆膜的化脓性炎症

- Empyema is a collection of pus in a hollow organ such as gallbladder or appendix

- 积脓发生于浆膜、胆囊和输卵管的化脓性炎症, 脓液则在浆膜、胆囊和输卵管腔内积存

- Phlegmonous inflammation is diffuse purulent inflammation in loose connective tissue. It often occurs in the skin, muscle and appendix, mainly caused by hemolytic streptococcus. The hyaluronidase secreted by Streptococcus degrades hyaluronic acid in loose connective tissue; the streptokinase secreted by Streptococcus dissolves fibrins, so bacteria easily spread

- 蜂窝织炎是疏松结缔组织的弥漫性化脓性炎症。常发生于皮肤、肌肉和阑尾, 主要由溶血性链球菌引起。链球菌分泌的透明质酸酶能降解疏松结缔组织中的透明质酸; 分泌的链激酶可溶解纤维素, 细菌易于扩散

- Abscess is localized collection of purulent inflammation accompanied by liquefactive necrosis. Abscess is characterized by cavity formation filling with necrosis and pus in subcutaneous or visceral organs. Abscess mainly caused by Staphylococcus aureus which could produce thrombin converting fibrinogen to fibers, so the lesions are more limited. Also, the bacteria have

- 脓肿为局限性化脓性炎症。主要特征是组织坏死, 形成充满脓液的腔。可发生于皮下和内脏, 主要由金黄葡萄球菌引起。金黄葡萄球菌可产生凝血酶, 使渗出的纤维蛋白原转变成纤维素, 则病变较局限; 具有层粘连蛋白受体, 使其容易通过血管壁而在远处产生迁徙性脓肿

laminin receptors could help going through the blood vessel wall to form migratory abscesses in the distance

- Hemorrhagic inflammations
  - Inflammation is characterized by large numbers of red blood cells in the exudate
  - It is common in epidemic hemorrhagic fever, leptospirosis and plague and other diseases

Consequences of acute inflammation

- Healing
- Transform to chronic inflammation
- Spread (direct, lymphatic and blood spread)
  - Bacteremia Bacteria enter the blood from local lesions. There are no symptoms of poisoning in the whole body, but bacteria can be found in the blood
  - Toxemia Toxic products or toxins of bacteria are into the blood with toxic symptoms
  - Septicemia After the bacteria enter the blood from the local lesions, they breed continuously and produce toxins causing systemic toxic symptoms
  - Pyemia Pyogenic organisms or bacteria in micro-thrombi spread

- 出血性炎症
  - 以渗出物中含有大量红细胞为特征的炎症
  - 常见于流行性出血热、钩端螺旋体病和鼠疫等疾病

急性炎症的结局

- 痊愈
- 转为慢性炎症
- 蔓延扩散 直接蔓延、淋巴道或血流播散
  - 菌血症 细菌由局部病灶入血，全身无中毒症状，但从血液中可查到细菌
  - 毒血症 细菌的毒性产物或毒素被进入血液，全身有中毒症状
  - 败血症 细菌由局部病灶入血后大量繁殖，并产生毒素，引起全身中毒症状
  - 脓毒败血症 化脓菌或微血栓中的细菌通过播散感染血流引起转

and infected blood flow giving rise to metastatic abscesses

移性脓肿所引起的败血症可进一步发展为脓毒败血症

Section 3　Chronic inflammation

第3节　慢性炎症

Conception

- Chronic inflammation is continuously response to against persistent injurious agents
- Chronic inflammation lasts for a long time mainly with proliferation lesions
- It is characterized by infiltrating of macrophages and lymphocytes

Chronic general inflammation

- The chronic inflammatory cells are including macrophages, lymphocytes, plasma cells, mast cells, etc.
- There are hyperplasia of various components including fibrous connective tissue, blood vessels, epithelial cells, glands and other parenchymal cells
- The persistent inflammatory agents or inflammatory cells will lead tissue damaged

Chronic granulomatous inflammation

- Inflammatory granuloma　is a special

概述

- 慢性炎症是对持续存在的损伤因子的反应

- 慢性炎症持续时间较长,以增生性病变为主
- 慢性炎症浸润的炎症细胞主要为巨噬细胞和淋巴细胞

普通慢性炎症

- 浸润细胞主要为巨噬细胞、淋巴细胞、浆细胞、肥大细胞等慢性炎症细胞
- 常伴有较为明显的纤维结缔组织、血管以及上皮细胞、腺体等实质细胞的增生

- 伴有组织的破坏,主要由持续的致炎因子或炎症细胞引起

慢性肉芽肿炎症

- 肉芽肿炎　是以肉芽肿形成为特点

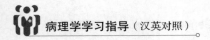

chronic inflammation characterized by
the formation of granulomas

- Granulomas are well-defined
  nodular lesions about 0.5～2 mm
  in diameter composed of localized
  proliferative macrophages and their
  developed cells
- Pathogenesis Some pathogens
  have strong resistance to phagocytosis
  and are not easy to be killed and
  degraded after being phagocytosed
  by macrophages. The morphology
  and function of macrophages changed
  after activation, the phagocytic
  function was significantly enhanced,
  and the morphology of itself was
  transformed into epithelioid cells or
  multinuclear giant cells
- Epithelioid cells are activated
  macrophages with abundant pale, foamy
  cytoplasm; they are called epithelial cells
  because of a superficial resemblance
  epithelial cell, epithelial cell appear to
  have enhanced ability to secret lysozyme
  and a variety of enzymes, but decreased
  phagocytic potential. Granulomas are
  usually surrounding by epithelial cells,
  lymphocyte, plasma cell, fibroblasts, etc.
- Types
  ○ Infective granuloma caused by
    infection with biological pathogens

的特殊慢性炎症

- 肉芽肿 是由巨噬细胞及其衍生细
  胞局部增生构成的境界清楚的结节
  状病灶，直径为0.5～2毫米

- 形成机制 一些病原物抵抗吞噬能
  力较强，被巨噬细胞吞噬后不易被杀
  伤降解，巨噬细胞激活后在形态和功
  能上均发生改变，其吞噬和消灭病原
  的能力显著增强，形态上转化为上皮
  样细胞或多核巨细胞

- 上皮样细胞 是活化的巨噬细胞，胞
  质丰富，呈苍白泡沫状，被称为上皮
  样细胞是因为其表面上与上皮细胞
  相似，上皮样细胞分泌溶菌酶和多种
  酶的能力增强，但吞噬潜能降低。肉
  芽肿通常周围被上皮样细胞、淋巴细
  胞、浆细胞、成纤维细胞等包围

- 类型
  ○ 感染性肉芽肿 由细菌、螺旋体、
    真菌、寄生虫等生物病原体感染

such as bacteria, spirochetes, fungi, parasites, etc. The mainly components are epithelioid cells and multinucleated giant cells

○ Granuloma of tuberculosis is composed of epithelioid cells, caseous necrosis, multinucleate giant cells (called Langhan's giant cell), lymphocytes, and fibroblasts

○ Foreign body granuloma represents nonimmune phagocytosis of foreign bodies without caseous necrosis. Granulomas caused by foreign bodies such as sutures, dust, etc. The granuloma is characterized by a foreign body surrounded by a large number of macrophages, multinucleate giant cells with foreign bodies (foreign body giant cell), fibroblasts and lymphocytes

○ Other granuloma unknown cause, such as sarcoid granuloma

引起的肉芽肿。主要成分是上皮样细胞和多核巨细胞

○ **结核肉芽肿** 由上皮样细胞、干酪样坏死、称为朗汉斯巨细胞的多核巨细胞、淋巴细胞和成纤维细胞组成

○ **异物肉芽肿** 指非免疫反应性吞噬作用，一般无干酪样坏死，是由缝线、粉尘等异物引起的肉芽肿。病变中心为异物，周围有大量巨噬细胞、异物巨细胞、成纤维细胞和淋巴细胞

○ **其他肉芽肿** 指原因不明肉芽肿如肉瘤样肉芽肿

顾昊煜　何妙侠

Chapter 5

Neoplasm

Section 1　Conception of neoplasm

Conception

- Neoplasm is new growth mass referred to abnormally cellular differentiation, maturation, and control of growth
- Neoplastic proliferation
  - It is monoclonal proliferation
  - The tumor is atypia and abnormal in morphology, mechanism, and function
  - The tumor proliferation is autonomous, uncoordinated, purposeless, and harmful to the body
- Non-neoplastic proliferation
  - It is reactive hyperplasia
  - Non-neoplastic proliferation is usually polyclonal with normal structure and function

第 5 章

肿瘤

第 1 节　肿瘤的概念

概述

- 肿瘤是机体的细胞异常增殖形成的新生物，常表现为异常细胞分化、成熟和生长控制

- 肿瘤性增殖
  - 肿瘤性增生一般为单克隆性
  - 肿瘤细胞具有异型性，在形态、代谢、功能均有异常

  - 肿瘤生长失去控制，无目的性，具有相对自主性；与机体不协调，对机体有害
- 非肿瘤性增殖
  - 是反应性增生
  - 非肿瘤性增生一般为多克隆性，细胞的结构和功能正常增生

○ The proliferation is under control, coordinated to the body's needs

○ 受到机体控制；与机体协调；符合机体需要

Section 2　Morphology of neoplasm

第2节　肿瘤的形态

🖋 Grossly feature

- **Numbers**　single, multiple
- **Size**　varies, occult carcinoma (< 1 cm)
- **Shape**　papillary, villous, cauliflower, polypods, nodular, lobulated, infiltrating, ulcerating, cystic
- **Color**　yellow, black, grey white
- **Consistency**　hard, soft
- **Margin between tumors and surrounding tissues**
  ○ Benign tumors usually have clear boundaries to surrounding tissues and may have a complete capsule
  ○ Malignant tumors generally have no capsule, often invade surrounding tissues, and the boundary is unclear

🖋 大体特征

- **肿瘤数目**　单发肿瘤、多发肿瘤
- **肿瘤大小**　差别很大，隐匿癌(<1厘米)
- **肿瘤形状**　乳头状、绒毛状、菜花状、息肉状、结节状、分叶状、浸润性、溃疡状、囊状
- **肿瘤的颜色**　黄色、黑色、灰白色
- **质地**　硬，软
- **肿瘤与周围组织关系**

  ○ 良性肿瘤通常与周围组织分界清晰，可有完整包膜

  ○ 恶性肿瘤一般无包膜，常侵入周围组织，边界不清

🖋 Morphological feature

- Microscopically, tumor tissue is composed of parenchyma and stroma
- Parenchyma is tumor cells which are the evidence for diagnosis of tumor atypia, differentiate, histological

🖋 形态特征

- 肿瘤组织是由肿瘤实质和间质构成的
- 肿瘤的实质由肿瘤细胞构成，是判断肿瘤细胞异型性、分化、组织学分类等的依据

classification and so on
- Stroma is composed of connective tissue, vessels and lymphocytes

Differentiation and atypia
- Tumor differentiation
  - The morphological and functional similarity of a tumor tissue to the original normal one
  - The morphology and function of the tumor are more like a certain normal one, the higher degree of the differentiation or well differentiation, the less similar to the normal tissue, the lower degree of the differentiation or poor differentiation
- Tumor atypia
  - The difference between tumor and corresponding normal tissue in architectural and cellular morphology
  - Architectural atypia of tumor the tumor tissue spatial structure formed by tumor cells is different from the corresponding normal tissue
  - Cellular atypia the difference between tumor cell and normal cells
    - The cellular atypia is including abnormal volume, size, and

- 肿瘤的间质由结缔组织、血管、数量不等的淋巴细胞构成

分化和异型性
- 肿瘤的分化
  - 肿瘤组织在形态和功能上与某种正常组织的相似之处

  - 肿瘤的组织形态和功能越是类似某种正常组织，分化程度越高或分化越好；与正常组织相似性越小，则分化程度越低或分化差

- 肿瘤的异型性
  - 肿瘤组织结构和细胞形态与相应的正常组织有不同程度的差异

  - 组织结构异型性 肿瘤细胞形成的组织结构，在空间排列方式上与相应正常组织的差异

  - 细胞异型性 肿瘤细胞与相应正常细胞之间的差异

    - 肿瘤细胞体积、大小和形态异常

shape of tumor cells

- The volume of tumor cell nuclei increases
- The nucleocytoplasmic ratio increases
- The size, shape and chromatin of nuclei vary greatly, that is called pleomorphism
- Nucleolus is obvious, large, and multiple
- Pathological mitotic figures are easily found

- 肿瘤细胞核的体积增大

- 核质比增高

- 细胞核的大小、形状和染色质差别较大,称核的多形性

- 核仁明显,体积大,数目增多

- 病理性核分裂象易见

Section 3　Tumor nomenclature and classification

第3节　肿瘤的命名和分类

Tumor nomenclature

- Benign tumor　tissue+ oma
- Malignant tumor
  - epithelial tissue + carcinoma
  - mesenchyme tissue+ sarcoma
- Special nomenclature
  - -blastoma, malignant
  - Leukemia, Seminoma
  - Melanoma, Malignant teratoma, malignant meningioma
  - Ewing's sarcoma, Hodgkin's lymphoma
  - Clear cell tumor

肿瘤的命名

- 良性肿瘤　组织+瘤
- 恶性肿瘤
  - 上皮组织　组织+癌
  - 间叶组织　组织+肉瘤
- 特殊的命名
  - 母细胞瘤,恶性肿瘤
  - 白血病,精原细胞瘤
  - 黑色素瘤,恶性畸胎瘤,恶性脑膜瘤
  - 尤因肉瘤,霍奇金淋巴瘤
  - 透明细胞瘤

○ Neurofibromatosis, lipomatosis, hemangiomatosis

○ Teratoma

○ Aneurysm, non-neoplasm

Tumor classification

- Benign tumor   compression
- Malignant tumor cachexia, paraneoplastic syndrome
- Borderline tumors are somewhere between benign and malignant in terms of morphology and biological behavior
- Tumor-like lesions are not true tumors, but their clinical presentation or histology resemble neoplastic lesions

Section 4 Tumor growth, invasion, and metastasis

Tumor growth

- Growth pattern
  ○ Expansive growth always shows well circumscribed mass, has capsule and compresses adjacent tissues
  ○ Exophytic growth papillary, polypoid growth on the skin and mucosa surface
  ○ Invasive growth tumor cells

○ 神经纤维瘤病，脂肪瘤病，血管瘤病

○ 畸胎瘤

○ 动脉瘤，非肿瘤

肿瘤的分类

- 良性肿瘤   压迫
- 恶性肿瘤   恶病质，副肿瘤综合征

- 交界性肿瘤   组织形态和生物学行为介于良恶性之间

- 瘤样病变   本身不是真性肿瘤，但其临床表现或组织形态类似肿瘤性病变

第4节 肿瘤的生长、扩散与转移

肿瘤的生长

- 肿瘤的生长方式
  ○ 膨胀性生长   肿瘤边界清楚，常有被膜，常压迫邻近组织
  ○ 外生性生长   在皮肤或体腔、黏膜表面的肿瘤呈乳头状、息肉状生长
  ○ 浸润性生长   肿瘤细胞浸润并破

infiltrating and destroy surrounding tissue including interstitial spaces, lymphatics, or blood vessels. The boundary between tumor and adjacent tissue is not clear

- Growth feature
  - Growth rate of tumors are different based on different double time, growth fraction and ratio of proliferation and death
  - Tumor angiogenesis is the feature of malignancy
- Progression and heterogeneity
  - Progression　There is an increase in invasiveness during the growth of malignant tumor
  - Heterogeneity　In the process of tumor growth, the progeny cells after many generations of division and reproduction may have different genetic or molecular changes, and difference in their growth rate, invasion ability, response to growth signals, sensitivity to anticancer drugs and so on

Tumor spread

- Invasion　Tumor cells infiltrate and destroy surrounding tissue including interstitial spaces, lymphatics, or blood vessels

坏周围组织（包括间质间隙、淋巴管或血管）。肿瘤与邻近组织界限不清

- 肿瘤的生长特征
  - 不同肿瘤的生长速度不同取决于其倍增时间，生长分数以及肿瘤增殖与死亡的比例等
  - 血管生成是恶性肿瘤的特征
- 肿瘤演进和异质化
  - 演进　恶性肿瘤生长过程中变得越来越具有侵袭性的现象
  - 异质化　肿瘤在生长过程中，经过许多代分裂繁殖产生的子代细胞，可出现不同的基因改变或其他大分子的改变，其生长速度、侵袭能力、对生长信号的反应、对抗癌药物的敏感性等方面都可以有差异

肿瘤扩散

- 浸润　肿瘤细胞长入并破坏周围组织包括组织间隙、淋巴管或血管

- **Direct spreading** Tumor cells infiltrate surrounding tissue continuously along the interstitial space or nerves, destroying adjacent organs or tissues with the growth of malignant tumors
- **Metastasis** Malignant tumor cells invade lymphatic vessels, blood vessels, or body cavities from the primary site, migrate to other sites, continue to grow, and form the same type of tumor
  - Lymphatic metastasis Neoplastic cells invade lymphatic vessels and follow the lymphatic flow to local lymph nodes (regional lymph nodes). It is the most common metastatic mode of epithelial malignancy (carcinoma)
  - Vascular metastasis Tumor cells can follow the blood stream to distant organs and continue to grow after tumor cells invade blood vessels. Tumor cells that invade the systemic circulation can enter the lung after passing through the right heart. The invaded tumor cells in the portal venous system reach liver first and form hepatic metastases. It is the most common metastatic mode of sarcoma
  - Transcoelomic metastasis Malignant tumor cells in the thoracic

- **直接蔓延** 随着恶性肿瘤不断长大，肿瘤细胞常常沿着组织间隙或神经束连续向周围浸润生长，破坏邻近器官或组织

- **转移** 恶性肿瘤细胞从原发部位侵入淋巴管、血管或体腔，迁徙到其他部位，继续生长，形成同样类型的肿瘤

  - **淋巴道转移** 肿瘤细胞侵入淋巴管，随淋巴流到达局部淋巴结（区域淋巴结）。淋巴道转移是上皮性恶性肿瘤（癌）最常见的转移方式

  - **血道转移** 肿瘤细胞侵入血管后，可随血流到达远处的器官，继续生长，形成转移瘤。侵入体循环的肿瘤细胞经右心到肺，侵入门静脉系统的肿瘤细胞，首先发生肝转移。血道转移是肉瘤最常见的转移模式

  - **种植性转移** 发生于胸腹腔等体腔内器官的恶性肿瘤，侵及器官

and abdominal cavity and cavity, when invading the surface of the organs, can fall off and be implanted on the surface of other organs in the body cavity like a seed, forming multiple metastatic tumors. It is the most common metastatic mode of gastric poorly carcinoma (Krukenberg tumor)

表面时，瘤细胞可以脱落，像播种一样种植在体腔其他器官的表面，形成多个转移性肿瘤。种植性转移是低分化胃癌最常见的转移模式（克鲁肯贝格瘤）

Section 5 & 6 Tumor grading, staging, and influence on patients

第5&6节 肿瘤分级与分期 肿瘤对机体的影响

Tumor grading and staging

- Tumor grade
  - grade 1   well differentiate
  - grade 2   medium differentiate
  - grade 3   poorly differentiate
- Tumor stage TNM
  - T primary tumor (1—4)
  - N lymph node metastasis (0—3)
  - M distance metastasis (0—1)
- Impacts of tumor on human body
  - Benign tumor   Just compress surrounding tissue
  - Malignant tumor   Cachexia, paraneoplastic syndrome
  - Borderline tumor   the behaviors are between benign and malignant

肿瘤分级与分期

- 肿瘤分级
  - 1级   高分化
  - 2级   中分化
  - 3级   低分化
- 肿瘤分期TNM
  - T 肿瘤原发灶（1—4）
  - N 淋巴结转移（0—3）
  - M 远处转移（0—1）
- 肿瘤对机体的影响
  - 良性肿瘤   少，压迫周围组织
  - 恶性肿瘤   恶病质，副肿瘤综合征
  - 交界性肿瘤   肿瘤生物学行为介于良恶性之间

○ Tumor-like lesions　It is not a true tumor

○ 瘤样病变　并非真正肿瘤

Section 7　Comparison of benign and malignant

第7节　良性肿瘤与恶性肿瘤

Comparison between benign and malignant tumor

区别

	Benign tumor	Malignant tumor
Differentiation	Well-differentiated, lower atypia	Loss of some normal differentiation either architecturally or cytoplasmically, higher atypia
Mitosis	None or few without pathologic mitosis	Many mitoses have pathologic mitosis
Growth Rate	Slow and may cease to grow	Rapid
Gross pattern	Expansile or exophytic growth, usually with capsule	Invasive or exophytic growth. The margin to adjacent tissue is not clear
Secondary changes	Little	Always with hemorrhage, necrosis and ulceration
Metastasis	None	Often have metastatic lesions
Recurrent	None or few	Easily recurrent
Influence to body	Mild, mainly compression or obstruction	Heavy, destruct tissue of primary and metastatic sites, with hemorrhage, necrosis, infection and cachexia

	良性肿瘤	恶性肿瘤
分化程度	分化好，异型性小	不同程度分化障碍或未分化，异型性大
核分裂象	无或少，不见病理性核分裂象	多，可见病理性核分裂象
生长速度	缓慢	较快
生长方式	膨胀或外生性生长，境界清，常有包膜	浸润或外生性生长，境界不清
继发改变	少见	常见，如出血、坏死、溃疡形成等
转移	不转移	可转移
复发	不复发或很少复发	易复发
对机体的影响	较小，主要为局部压迫或阻塞	较大，破坏原发部位和转移部位的组织；坏死、出血，合并感染；恶病质

Section 8　Common tumors

- Epithelial benign tumor
  - Papilloma
  - Adenoma
    - Tubular adenoma
    - Villous adenoma
    - Tubulovillous adenoma
    - Cystadenoma
- Epithelial malignant tumor
  - Squamous cell carcinoma
  - Adenocarcinoma
  - Basal cell carcinoma
  - Urothelial carcinoma
- Mesenchymal benign tumor
  - Lipoma
  - Hemangioma
  - Lymphangioma
  - Leiomyoma
  - Chondroma
- Mesenchyme malignant tumor
  - Liposarcoma
  - Rhabdomyosarcoma
  - Leiomyosarcoma
  - Angiosarcoma
  - Osteosarcoma
  - Chondrosarcoma
  - Lymphoma
- Neuroectoblastoid tumor
  - Glioma

第8节　常见肿瘤

- 上皮源性良性肿瘤
  - 乳头状瘤
  - 腺瘤
    - 管状腺瘤
    - 绒毛状腺瘤
    - 管状-绒毛状腺瘤
    - 囊腺瘤
- 上皮源性恶性肿瘤
  - 鳞状细胞癌
  - 腺癌
  - 基底细胞癌
  - 尿路上皮癌
- 间叶源性良性肿瘤
  - 脂肪瘤
  - 血管瘤
  - 淋巴管瘤
  - 平滑肌瘤
  - 软骨瘤
- 间叶源性恶性肿瘤
  - 脂肪肉瘤
  - 横纹肌肉瘤
  - 平滑肌肉瘤
  - 血管肉瘤
  - 骨肉瘤
  - 软骨肉瘤
  - 淋巴瘤
- 神经外胚叶肿瘤
  - 胶质瘤

- ○ Retinoblastoma
- ○ Melanoma
- Other tumors
  - ○ Carcinosarcoma Carcinoma + Sarcoma
  - ○ Teratoma Multi-ectoderm tumor

- ○ 视网膜母细胞瘤
- ○ 黑色素瘤
- 其他肿瘤
  - ○ 癌肉瘤 含癌和肉瘤两种成分
  - ○ 畸胎瘤 含多个胚层分化的肿瘤

 ## Comparison between carcinoma and sarcoma

	Carcinoma	Sarcoma
Tissue differentiation	Epithelium	Mesenchymal tissue
Incidence	More common. Nine time as much as that of sarcoma. More often in adult over forties	Less common. Some types more often occur in children and youngers, some in older
Gross features	Hard, gray-white color	Softer, moist, and fleshy
Microscopical features	Cancerous cell nests. Distinct demarcation between parenchyma and stroma	Tumor cells arrangement diffusely. Parenchyma and stroma mixed without demarcation
Reticular fiber	Around the cancerous nests, without among the cells	Among the tumor cells
Metastasis	Always by lymphatic vessels	Often via blood vessels

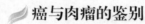 ## 癌与肉瘤的鉴别

	癌	肉瘤
组织分化	上皮组织	间叶组织
发病率	较高，约为肉瘤9倍，多见于40岁以后成人	较低，有些类型多见于年轻人或儿童，有些类型多见于中老年人
大体特点	质硬，色灰白	质软，色灰红，鱼肉状
组织学特点	多形成癌巢，实质间质分界清楚，纤维组织常有增生	肉瘤细胞多弥漫分布，实质间质分界不清，间质血管丰富，纤维组织少
网状纤维	见于癌巢周围，癌细胞间无网状纤维	肉瘤细胞间多有网状纤维
转移	多经淋巴道	多经血道

Section 9 Precancerous diseases, dysplasia and carcinoma *in situ*

Precancerous diseases (lesions)

- **Definition** Although certain diseases (lesions) are not malignant tumors themselves, they have the potential to develop into malignant tumors, and patients are increased at risk of developing corresponding malignant tumors
- Common precancerous diseases
  ○ Colonic adenoma
  ○ Atypical ductal hyperplasia of breast
  ○ Atrophic gastritis and intestinal metaplasia
  ○ Chronic ulcerative colitis
  ○ Skin chronic ulcer
  ○ Leukoplakia

Dysplasia

- Dysplasia is an abnormality of both differentiation and maturation of cells. Atypical hyperplasia associated with tumorigenesis, in which cells proliferate with atypia
- The cellular changes are made up of pleomorphic cells, loss of polarity,

第9节 癌前疾病 异型增生 原位癌

癌前疾病（病变）

- **定义** 某些疾病（病变）虽然本身不是恶性肿瘤,但具有发展为恶性肿瘤的潜能,患者发生相应恶性肿瘤的风险增加

- **常见癌前病变**
  ○ 大肠腺瘤
  ○ 乳腺导管上皮不典型增生
  ○ 萎缩性胃炎伴肠上皮化生
  ○ 慢性溃疡性结肠炎
  ○ 皮肤慢性溃疡
  ○ 黏膜白斑

异型增生

- 异型增生指细胞在分化和成熟的异常。与肿瘤形成相关的非典型增生,细胞增生并出现异型性

- 肿瘤变化包括细胞多形性,极向消失,核染色质高,核分裂象易见,但无

hyperchromatic nuclei, increased mitosis, but no invasion

浸润

Carcinoma in situ (CIS)

- Carcinoma in situ is the earliest stage of carcinoma
- It denotes carcinomatous changes are just limited in the epithelium without any evidence of the invasion and has not breakthrough basement membrane

原位癌

- 异常增生的细胞在形态和功能上与癌细胞相似
- 常累及上皮全层，但没有突破基底膜向下浸润

Intraepithelial neoplasia (IN)

- The continuous process of epithelial dysplasia to carcinoma *in situ*, divided into low-grade and high-grade intraepithelial neoplasia

上皮内瘤变

- 上皮从异型增生到原位癌这一连续的过程，分低级别和高级别上皮内瘤变

Section 10　Molecular mechanism of tumorigenesis

第10节　肿瘤发生的分子机制

Oncogene activity

- Point mutation
- Gene amplification
- Chromosomal rearrangement

癌基因活化

- 点突变
- 基因扩增
- 染色体重排

Tumor suppressor gene inactivity

- *RB* gene inactivity
- *p53* gene mutation
- *NF1* gene mutation

抑癌基因失活

- *RB* 基因失活
- *p53* 基因突变
- *NF1* 基因突变

- *APC* gene inactivity
- *p16* gene inactivity
- *VHL gene* mutation

Multi-step of malignant transformation

Colonic adenocarcinoma

- *APC* mutation—DNA methylation—*Ras* mutation—DCC loss—*p53* mutation—other mutation
- Normal—hyperplasia—early adenoma—medium adenoma—later adenoma—carcinoma—metastasis

Section 11&12   Environmental and genetic factors of tumorigenesis

Chemicals

- PAH polycyclic aromatic hydrocarbon   Lung cancer
- Aromatic amines   Bladder carcinoma
- Nitrite   Gastric carcinoma
- Mycotoxins Aflatoxin B   Hepatic cell carcinoma
- Alkylation agents   Leukemia

Physical agents

- Ultral violet   Skin carcinoma, melanoma

- *APC*基因失活
- *p16*基因失活
- *VHL* 基因突变

多步癌变机制

大肠腺癌为例

- *APC*基因突变—DNA甲基化—*Ras*基因突变—DCC失活—*p53*基因突变—其他基因突变
- 正常黏膜—增生—早期腺瘤—中期腺瘤—晚期腺瘤—腺癌—转移

第 11&12 节   环境遗传致瘤因素

化学物

- 多环芳烃   肺癌
- 芳香胺类   膀胱癌
- 亚硝酸胺   胃癌
- 真菌毒素   黄曲霉毒素 B 肝癌
- 烷化剂   白血病

物理因素

- 紫外线   皮肤癌和黑色素瘤

- Ionizing radiation　Leukemia

Biological agents

- HPV　Human papilloma virus Cervix carcinoma
- E B V 　 E p s t e i n - B a r r v i r u s Nasopharyngeal carcinoma
- HBV　Hepatitis virus B Hepatic carcinoma
- HTLV-1　RNA virus T cell leukemia

- HP　H. Pylori Gastric carcinoma or lymphoma

Genetic factors

- Genetic tumor syndrome
  ○ Autosomal dominant
  ○ Autosomal
- Familial cancer
  ○ Breast cancer
  ○ Gastrointestinal cancer

- 电离辐射　白血病

生物因素

- 人类乳头状瘤病毒　宫颈癌

- EB病毒　鼻咽癌

- 乙型肝炎病毒　肝癌

- 人类T细胞白血病病毒　T细胞白血病
- 幽门螺杆菌　胃癌和淋巴瘤

遗传因素

- 遗传肿瘤综合征
  ○ 常染色体显性
  ○ 常染色体隐性
- 家族性肿瘤
  ○ 乳腺癌
  ○ 胃肠癌

顾昊煜　何妙侠

Systemic pathology
病理学各论

Chapter 6

Diseases of Cardiovascular System

第6章

心血管系统疾病

Section 1　Atherosclerosis

🌿 Conception

- Arteriosclerosis is including atherosclerosis, monckeberg medial sclerosis and arteriolosclerosis
- Atherosclerosis (ATH) is a disease involving large and medium arteries with lipid deposition and vascular wall stenosis

🌿 Etiology and Pathogenesis

- Risk factors
  - Hyperlipidemia High cholesterol, triglyceride. Oxidized LDL
  - Hypertension
  - Cigarette Smoking
  - Diabetes Mellitus
  - Genetic factors
  - Age, Gender, Obesity
- Pathogenesis
  - Hypothesis of lipid substance

第1节　动脉粥样硬化

🌿 概述

- **动脉硬化**　包括动脉粥样硬化,动脉中层硬化,细动脉硬化

- **动脉粥样硬化**　累及大中型动脉,以脂质沉积和血管壁硬化为特征

🌿 病因与病机

- 危险因素
  - 高脂血症　胆固醇和/或甘油三酯
  - 高血压
  - 吸烟
  - 糖尿病
  - 遗传因素
  - 年龄,性别,肥胖度
- 发病机制
  - 脂质渗入学说

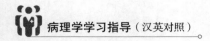
deposition　High LDL ox-LDL

    ○ Hypothesis of reaction to vascular injury

    ○ Hypothesis of arterial smooth muscle cells (SMC)

    ○ Hypothesis of chronic inflammation

Pathological changes

- Fatty streak
  - Reversible　commonly in the posterior wall of the aorta and the opening of the branch
  - Grossly　earliest lesion, yellow flat spot, or streak
  - Microscopically　Foamy cells aggregation
- Fibrous plaque
  - Irreversible
  - Grossly　yellow-white elevation on the intimal surface of the artery
  - Microscopically　Fibrotic capsule, foamy cell
- Atheromatous plaque
  - Irreversible
  - Grossly　grey yellow plaque, in cut section, the center of the plaque consists of semisolid yellow material like porridge
  - Microscopically　the three zones are recognizable of Fibrous capsule, foamy cells and lipid pool. Needle-

○ 损伤应答学说

○ 动脉平滑肌细胞学说

○ 慢性炎症学说

病理变化

- 脂纹期
  - 可逆　常见于主动脉后壁及分支开口处

  - 肉眼　肉眼可见的最早改变，黄色点状或条纹
  - 镜下　泡沫细胞

- 纤维斑块期
  - 不可逆
  - 肉眼　瓷白色突出于表面

  - 镜下　纤维帽及泡沫细胞

- 粥样斑块期
  - 不可逆
  - 肉眼　黄色粥糜样

  - 镜下　纤维帽，泡沫细胞，脂质池，可见胆固醇结晶

shaped cholesterol crystals are commonly present in the lipid pool

- Complicated lesions
  - Hemorrhage
  - Plaque rupture
  - Thrombosis most common complication
  - Dystrophic calcification
  - Aneurysm
  - Narrow of artery

Pathological changes of main arteries

- Atherosclerosis in aorta
  - It is commonly in the posterior wall of the aorta and the opening of the branch, especially in abdominal aorta
  - Aneurysm is formed and easily broken
- Atherosclerosis in kidney
  - It is commonly in the opening of the kidney arterial branch and proximal of aorta
  - The lesions are multiple irregular infarctions and scars causing ATH related atrophy of kidney
- Atherosclerosis in extremities
  - It is commonly in lower limb caused by ATH in artery, femoral artery, and shin artery
  - The patients always present intermittent claudication or gangrene of limb

- 继发性病变
  - 斑块内出血
  - 斑块破裂
  - 血栓形成

  - 营养不良性钙化
  - 动脉瘤形成
  - 血管狭窄

主要动脉病理变化

- 主动脉粥样硬化
  - 常见于主动脉后壁及其分支开口处，以腹主动脉最为严重

  - 常形成动脉瘤，且易破裂
- 肾动脉粥样硬化
  - 常见于肾动脉开口处及主动脉近侧端

  - 病变常导致多个梗死灶及疤痕形成，形成动脉粥样硬化性固缩肾

- 四肢动脉粥样硬化
  - 常见于下肢，多由腘动脉、股动脉和胫动脉粥样硬化引起

  - 患者常出现间歇性跛行和下肢坏疽

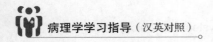

- Atherosclerosis in mesentery
  - It will cause intestinal infraction and obstruction
  - The patient always complains of abdominal pain

- Atherosclerosis in brain
  - ATH is commonly seen in the begin of cervical artery, basal artery, cerebral middle artery, Willis circle
  - Cerebral atrophy, infraction and aneurysm are common lesions
  - Cerebral hemorrhage usually caused by aneurysm broken
- Coronary atherosclerosis
  - ATH is most common seen in anterior descending branch of heart coronary
  - Coronary atherosclerosis always causes coronary heart diseases (CHD)

Coronary heart diseases (CHD)
- Pathological changes
  - **Grossly** The lesions usually located near to the ventricular wall like moon shape. Coronary artery lumen become narrow
  - **Microscopically** ATH typical morphology with fibrous capsule, foamy cells and lipid pool, and the

- 肠系膜动脉粥样硬化
  - 常引起肠梗死和肠梗阻

  - 病变常导致多个梗死灶及瘢痕形成，形成动脉粥样硬化性固缩肾患者常出现腹痛
- 脑动脉粥样硬化
  - 常见于颈动脉起始处、基底动脉、大脑中动脉和大脑动脉环

  - 病变常表现为脑萎缩、脑梗死和脑动脉瘤形成
  - 动脉瘤破裂是引起脑出血

- 冠状动脉粥样硬化
  - 常见于冠状动脉前降支

  - 冠状动脉粥样硬化常引起冠状动脉性心脏病（冠心病）

冠心病
- 病理改变
  - **大体** 冠状动脉血管壁靠近心室壁侧出现新月形病变，管腔狭窄

  - **镜下** 呈现典型动脉粥样硬化形态学表现如纤维帽，泡沫细胞和脂质池，并可见继发性病变

secondary lesions might be found

- Obstructive degrees of coronary lumen
  - Grade 1 ≤ 25%
  - Grade 2 26% ～ 50%
  - Grade 3 51% ～ 75%
  - Grade 4 ＞ 75%
- Pathological types of CHD
  - Angina pectoris is characterized episodic ischemic cardiac pain not associated with infracts
    - Stable angina pectoris Slightly, inducing by myocardial workload increase such as angry or after big dinner
    - Instable angina pectoris Severe, no inducer
    - Variant angina pectoris (Prinzmetal) occurs at rest without relate to myocardial work, possibly caused by coronary artery muscle spasm
  - Myocardial infarction (MI)
    - Grossly subendocardial, multi-foci, transmural infarction
    - Microscopically coagulation necrosis
    - Locations of MI
      A 50% of left coronary artery anterior descending branch including left ventricle anterior

- 冠状动脉狭窄程度

  - 1级 ≤ 25%
  - 2级 26% ～ 50%
  - 3级 51% ～ 75%
  - 4级 ＞ 75%
- 冠心病病理类型
  - 心绞痛 发作性心肌缺血性疼痛,与心梗无关

    - 稳定心绞痛 较轻,与心肌工作负荷加重有关,如生气,饱食

    - 不稳定心绞痛 较重,无诱因

    - 变异型心绞痛 休息时发病,与心肌负荷无关

  - 心肌梗塞
    - 大体 心内膜下、多灶性、穿壁性梗死
    - 镜下 凝固性坏死

    - 部位
      A 50%左前降支包括左心室前壁、心尖部和室间隔前2/3

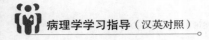

wall; heart apex; anterior 2/3 of ventricular septum

B 30% of right coronary artery including left ventricle posterior wall; right ventricle; back 1/3 of ventricular septum

C 20% of left circumflex branch including left ventricle posterior wall

- Complication of MI including Heart failure, cardiogenic shock, cardiac rupture, ventricular aneurysm, mural thrombus, pericarditis, and arrhythmia
○ Myocardial fibrosis
  - Chronic ischemic heart disease caused by persistent or recurrent ischemia and hypoxia of myocardial fibers, and coronary artery stenosis
○ Sudden coronary death
  - Acute coronary ischemia and severe arrhythmia caused by blood flow interruption

B 30% 右冠状动脉包括左心室后壁、右心室和室间隔后 1/3

C 20% 左旋支左心室后壁

- 并发症
  心力衰竭，心脏破裂，心源性休克，室性动脉瘤，附壁血栓，心包炎和心律失常
○ 心肌纤维化
  - 冠状动脉狭窄致心肌纤维持续性或反复性缺血、缺氧所致的慢性缺血性心脏病
○ 冠心病猝死
  - 冠状动脉急性缺血，血流中断引起严重心律失常所致

Section 2   Hypertension

Conception

- Hypertension refers to a persistent increase in arterial blood pressure in

第 2 节　高血压

概述

- 高血压是指体循环动脉血压持续升高

the systemic circulation

- It is a common clinical syndrome that can lead to neoplastic, cerebral, renal, and vascular changes
- Adult normal blood pressure
  ○ Systolic blood pressure < 120 mmHg (16 kPa)

    and
  ○ Diastolic blood pressure < 80 mmHg (10.6 kPa)
- Borderline blood pressure
  ○ Systolic blood pressure 120 ～ 139 mmHg

    And /or
  ○ Diastolic blood pressure 80 ～ 90 mmHg
- Adult hypertension
  ○ Systolic blood pressure ≥ 140 mmHg (18.6 kPa)

    And /or
  ○ Diastolic blood pressure ≥ 90 mmHg (12 kPa)
- Classifications
  ○ Primary hypertension   No definitely reason
    - Benign   Essential hypertension more than 95%
    - Malignant   Accelerated hypertension
  ○ Secondary hypertension   Based on some disease

- 高血压是一种可导致心、脑、肾和血管改变的常见临床综合征

- 成人正常血压
  ○ 收缩压 < 120 毫米汞柱（16千帕）

    和
  ○ 舒张压 < 80 毫米汞柱（10.6千帕）

- 临界血压
  ○ 收缩压　120 ～ 139 毫米汞柱

    和/或
  ○ 舒张压　80 ～ 90 毫米汞柱

- 成人高血压
  ○ 收缩压 ≥ 140 毫米汞柱（18.6千帕）

    和/或
  ○ 舒张压 ≥ 90 毫米汞柱（12千帕）

- 分类
  ○ 原发性高血压　无明确原因
    - 良性　特发性高血压占95%
    - 恶性　急进性高血压
  ○ 继发性高血压　继发于某些病变

Etiology and Pathogenesis

- Risk factors
  - Genetic factors　Probably polygenetic changes
  - Dietary habits　High salt diet, Obesity, Drink
  - Social and mentally factors Stressful
  - Lack of exercise
  - Neural endocrine factors Sympathetic nerves activity
- Pathogenesis
  - Genetic mechanism
  - Renin-angiotensin-aldosterone System (RAAS) activate
  - Sympathetic nerves stress
  - Disorder of endothelial function
  - Anti-Insulins
  - Vascular remodeling

Primary hypertension

Stages

- Functional disorder
  - Early stage　There are no microscopic changes
  - Mechanism　Vasoconstriction by smooth muscle contraction
  - Clinical manifestation Asymptomatically, occasional headache, dizziness, elevated blood pressure, etc.

病因与病机

- 危险因素
  - 遗传因素　可能是多基因遗传
  - 饮食习惯　如高盐饮食、肥胖、饮酒
  - 社会心理　精神压力大
  - 缺乏锻炼
  - 神经内分泌因素　交感神经兴奋
- 病理机制
  - 遗传机制
  - 肾素-血管紧张素-醛固酮系统活化
  - 交感神经系统紧张
  - 血管内皮功能紊乱
  - 胰岛素抵抗
  - 血管结构重建

原发性高血压

分期

- 功能紊乱期
  - 早期　无镜下变化
  - 机制　血管间断性收缩
  - 临床表现　为头痛、头晕、高血压等

- Treatment Exercise could restore blood pressure to the normal range, but it is often ignored
- Artery lesion
  - Involving small arterial vessels
  - Pathological changes Thicken wall and narrow lumen
  - Causes The sustained vasoconstriction leading blood vessel media thickening and hyaline degeneration, and intimal fibrosis called hyaline arteriolosclerosis, media muscle hypertrophy and permeability of blood vessels increased
  - Clinical manifestation blood pressure increasing, irreversible
  - Therapeutic approach continuous antihypertension treatment
- Organ changes
  - Heart
    Hypertensive heart disease
    - Mainly involving the left ventricle
    - Early compensatory concentric cardiac hypertrophy
    - Lately incompensatory eccentric cardiohypertrophy
    - Severely heart failure
  - Kidney
    - Primary granular atrophy of the kidney
    - Grossly

- 治疗 锻炼可以恢复,但常不被重视
- 动脉病变期
  - 主要累及 细小动脉
  - 病理特点 厚壁腔小
  - 原因 持续性的血管收缩导致血管中膜变厚玻璃样变和内膜纤维化,被称为细小动脉玻璃样变性,中膜平滑肌萎缩和血管通透性增加
  - 临床表现 血压升高,不可逆性
  - 应对方法 持续抗高血压药物治疗
- 内脏病变期
  - 心脏
    高血压性心脏病
    - 主要累及 左心室
    - 早期 代偿性向心性肥大
    - 后期 失代偿性离心性肥大
    - 严重 导致心衰
  - 肾脏病变
    - 原发性颗粒性固缩肾
    - 大体

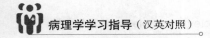

Bilateral kidneys small, light and hard

双侧肾 小、轻、硬

Surface full of homogeneous fine granular

表面 充满均匀的细颗粒

Cutting surface renal cortical atrophy

切面 见肾皮质萎缩

Cortico-medullary boundary unclear

皮髓质边界 不清

- Microscopically

- 镜下

Concave due to renal afferent arteriolar hyalinosis, involved nephron atrophy and fibrosis

凹陷 是由于肾小球小动脉玻璃样变累及肾单位萎缩和纤维化

Convex due to intact nephron compensatory dilatation

突起 是由于完整肾单位代偿性扩张

○ Brain

○ 脑部病变

- Hypertensive encephalopathy (brain edema)

- 高血压脑病（脑水肿）

Brain small arterial sclerosis and spasm, ischemia, cerebral edema, patients with headache, dizziness, vertigo, vomiting and other signs

大脑小动脉硬化及痉挛，缺血，脑水肿时，患者表现为头痛，头晕，目眩，恶心等症状

- Softening of brain microinfarction

- 脑梗死

- Cerebral hemorrhage could be severe

- 脑出血 严重

○ Retina

○ 高血压性视网膜病变

- Arteriolosclerosis of retinal central artery

- 视网膜中央动脉小动脉硬化

Malignant hypertension

恶性高血压

- Pathologic change

- 病理变化

○ Hyperplastic arteriolosclerosis

○ 增生性动脉硬化

- ○ Necrotizing arteriolitis
- Involve organs
  - ○ Kidney
  - ○ Brain
  - ○ Retina
- Clinical features
  - ○ Higher blood pressure (＞230/130 mmHg)
  - ○ Hypertensive encephalopathy
  - ○ Brain hemorrhage
  - ○ Renal failure

Section 3　Rheumatism

Conception

- Rheumatism is associated with group A Beta-hemolytic streptococcus infection
- It is seen in 5～15 years of age and involves connective tissue and blood vessels throughout the body such as heart, joints, skin, and central nervous system
- The clinical manifestations are including fever, elevated anti-O antibody, erythrocyte sedimentation rate, and white blood cells, and prolonged PR interval of electrocardiogram

The basic pathological changes

- Alterative and exudative phase
  - ○ Lasting for 1 month

- ○ 坏死性动脉炎
- 主要累及
  - ○ 肾
  - ○ 脑
  - ○ 视网膜
- 临床表现
  - ○ 血压急剧升高（＞230/130毫米汞柱）
  - ○ 高血压脑病
  - ○ 脑出血
  - ○ 肾衰

第3节　风湿病

概述

- 与A组乙型溶血性链球菌感染有关

- 见于5～15岁，累及全身结缔组织和血管，常见于心脏、关节、皮肤和中枢神经系统

- 临床表现为发热、抗O抗体，血沉、白细胞升高，心电图PR间期延长

基本病变

- 变质渗出期
  - ○ 持续1个月

- Matrix mucoid degeneration
- Fibrinous necrosis of collagen fibers
- Serous fluid effusion, lymphocytes, plasma cells and monocytes

- Proliferative phase (granulomatous phase)
  - Lasting for 2 to 3 months
  - Aschoff body the shape like slightly fusiform. It consists of groups of rheumatoid cells that accumulate in fibrinoid necrosis foci, infiltrated by a small amount of lymphoid and plasma cells, and interstitial myxoid degeneration
- Fibrous phase
  - Lasting 3 to 4 months
  - The necrosis disappears and rheumatic cells changed to fibroblast cells and fibrocytes, then to collagen fibers, then hyaline change and eventually into scar tissue
  - If the lesion involves the serosa, it always shows serous and fibrinous exudation

Rheumatic pathological changes in the organs

Rheumatic heart disease

- Rheumatic endocarditis
  - The valves of the left side of heart

- 基质黏液样变性
- 胶原纤维纤维素样坏死

- 浆液、淋巴、浆细胞及单核细胞渗出
- 增生期或肉芽肿期

  - 持续2～3个月
  - 阿绍夫小体 由成群风湿细胞聚集于纤维素样坏死灶内，伴少量淋巴、浆细胞浸润，间质黏液样变

- 纤维化期
  - 持续3～4个月
  - 坏死吸收，风湿细胞变成成纤维细胞、纤维细胞，最后变成瘢痕组织

  - 如果病变累及浆膜，表现为浆液、纤维素性炎

风湿病各器官病变

风湿性心脏病

- 风湿性心内膜炎
  - 左心瓣膜易累及且病变严重，二

are affected more often and more severely, the mitral valve more than the aortic

尖瓣较主动脉瓣易受损

- Involved valves show edema and denudation of the lining endocardium

○ 受损瓣膜水肿、瓣膜闭锁缘受损

- In areas of maximal trauma at the line of apposition of the free edge of the valve

○ 瓣膜闭锁缘故的广泛分布单行排列的病变

- Rheumatic vegetations are composed of platelet-fibrin thrombi do not become detached as emboli

○ 风湿病赘生物是由血小板和纤维素构成的血栓,不容易脱落

- McCallum plaque valvular stenosis or regurgitation causes focal endocardial thickening

○ **马氏斑** 指由于瓣膜硬化导致血流反流引起局部心内膜增厚的现象

- Rheumatic myocarditis
  - It is characterized by the presence of numerous of Aschoff bodies in the myocardium
  - Involving left atrium, left ventricles, left atrial septa
  - Aschoff bodies locate in interstitial perivascular area
  - There occur arrhythmias, tachycardia, dilation of heart, myocardial fibrosis

- **风湿性心肌炎**
  ○ 特征性改变是心肌间出现多个阿绍夫小体

  ○ 累及左心房、左心室及左房间隔

  ○ 风湿小体位于心肌间质小血管旁

  ○ 常出现心律失常、心动过速、心脏扩大和心肌纤维化

- Rheumatic pericarditis
  - It is mainly involved epicardial layer called cor villosum
  - There are more serous fluid leads to pericardial effusion belong to serous or fibrinous inflammation
  - Result little pericardial effusion

- **风湿性心包炎**
  ○ 常累及心外膜引起典型绒毛心

  ○ 心包常有浆液渗出,属于浆液纤维素性炎

  ○ **结局** 渗出少,影响小;渗出多形

can be absorbed; more effusion leads adhesive pericarditis

成心包积液，渗出多易形成心包粘连

- Rheumatic arthritis
  - It is serous exudation and less affecting on joins
  - "Bite the heart, Kick the joint"
- Rheumatic skin lesion
  - Annular erythema (exudative lesion)
  - Subcutaneous nodules (hyperplasia)
- Rheumatic arteritis
  - Involve middle and large arterials
- CNS lesion (chorea)
  - Involve 5 ~ 12 year old girl
  - Involve extrapyramidal system, lead to chorea

- 风湿性关节炎
  - 常有浆液性渗出，对关节影响小
  - "扎心敲关"
- 风湿性皮肤病
  - 环状红斑（渗出性病变）
  - 皮下结节（增生）
- 风湿性动脉炎
  - 累及大中型动脉
- 中枢神经系统病变（舞蹈症）
  - 累及5～12岁小女孩
  - 常累及锥体外系，导致舞蹈症

Section 4　Subacute infective endocarditis

第4节　亚急性感染性心内膜炎

Etiology and Pathogenesis

- Caused by streptococcus viridans with weak pathogenicity
- Involving multiple valves with basic disease (such as rheumatic endocarditis)
- Infective route bacteria from the local infectious lesion enter the blood and then to heart valves

病因与病机

- 由致病力弱的草绿色链球菌引起，常累及多个瓣膜
- 累及基础病变（例如风湿性心内膜炎）的有瓣膜
- 细菌由原发感染部位经血传播至瓣膜

Pathologic changes

- Characterized　by the formation of

病理变化

- **特点**　瓣膜赘生物形成

vegetations on the valves

- Grossly There are large, grey, and yellowish irregularly arranged vegetations involving endocardium and easily drop off
- Microscopically mixed thrombus containing bacteria
- Results Often lead to severe valvular disease
- Treatment Antibiotics

- **大体** 角度大且呈污秽、灰黄色的赘生物,易脱落

- **镜下** 包含细菌的混合血栓

- **结局** 易导致严重的瓣膜疾病

- **治疗** 使用抗生素治疗

Comparison between rheumatic endocarditis and subacute infective endocarditis

风湿性心内膜炎与亚急性心内膜炎比较

	Rheumatic endocarditis	Infective endocarditis
Etiology	Group A B Hemolytic streptococcus (allergic disease)	Bacterial, fungal, rickettsia caused by inflammatory diseases
Involved valve	Mitral valve, Aortic valve	Mitral valve, Aortic valve
Vegetation features	**Grossly** gray, transparent, single line, diameter 1～2 mm, do not fall off **Microscopically** Platelets, fibrin	**Grossly** green, large, polypoid, cauliflower, brittle. Easy to fall off **Microscopically** platelets, necrosis, bacteria and inflammatory cells
Results and complications	valve thickening, harden, curling, shortening, chronic valvular disease	valve rupture, perforation, cord rupture, chronic valvular disease, sepsis, death

	风湿性心内膜炎	感染性心内膜炎
病因	A组乙型溶血性链球菌(变态反应性疾病)	病原微生物(细菌、真菌、立克次体引起的炎症性疾病)
主要累及瓣膜	二尖瓣、主动脉瓣	二尖瓣、主动脉瓣
赘生物特点	**大体**:灰白,半透明,单行串珠样,直径1～2毫米,质软,不易脱落 **镜下**:血小板、纤维素	**大体**:灰黄浅绿色,体积大,息肉状、菜花状,松脆,易脱落 **镜下**:血小板、坏死、细菌菌落、炎细胞
结局及并发症	瓣膜增厚、变硬、卷曲、缩短、慢性心瓣膜病	瓣膜破裂、穿孔,腱索断裂,慢性心瓣膜病,脓毒血症,死亡

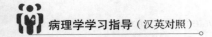

Section 5　Valvular heart disease

🖋 Etiology

- Rheumatic endocarditis, infective endocarditis
- Aortic atherosclerosis, syphilitic aortitis
- Congenital valve abnormalities, valvular calcification

🖋 Types

Valvular stenosis and/or Valvular insufficiency

- Mitral stenosis
  - Hemodynamic changes　involving diastolic phase
  - Mitral stenosis→left ventricular perfusion reduce →left atrial congestion and dilatation →pulmonary congestion→ pulmonary edema, pulmonary artery high pressure→ right ventricular hypertrophy and dilatation→right atrial hypertrophy and expansion→ right heart failure
  - X-ray　Pear shaped heart
  - Auscultation　Apical diastolic rumbling murmur of heart
  - Signs　Pulmonary congestion, dyspnea, cyanosis, bloody foam sputum

第5节　心瓣膜病

🖋 病因

- 风湿性心内膜炎,感染性心内膜炎
- 主动脉粥样硬化,梅毒性主动脉炎
- 先天性瓣膜异常,瓣膜钙化

🖋 类型

瓣膜狭窄和/或关闭不全

- 二尖瓣狭窄
  - 血流动力学　累及心脏舒张期
  - 二尖瓣口狭窄→左室灌注不足,左房淤血→左房肥大扩张→肺淤血水肿、肺动脉高压→右室肥大扩张→右房肥大扩张→大循环淤血
  - X线　梨形心
  - 听诊　心尖区舒张期隆隆样杂音
  - 症状　肺淤血表现为呼吸困难、发绀、血性泡沫痰,右心衰竭表现为颈静脉怒张,肝脾肿大,下肢

- Mitral insufficiency
  - Hemodynamic changes involving systolic phase
  - Mitral insufficiency→part of left ventricular blood reflux into left atrium→left atrial hypertrophy and dilatation→ left ventricular hypertrophy and dilatation → pulmonary congestion and pulmonary artery high pressure→right ventricular hypertrophy and dilatation, →right atrial hypertrophy and expansion → right heart failure
  - X-ray Spherical shaped heart because of left atrium and ventricular hypertrophy
  - Auscultation Apical systolic blowing murmur of heart
  - Signs Pulmonary congestion, dyspnea, cyanosis, hepatosplenomegaly, lower extremity edema
- Aortic stenosis
  - Hemodynamic changes involving systolic phase
  - Aortic stenosis→left ventricular injection hindered→left ventricular concentric and eccentric hypertrophy → left atrial hypertrophy and dilatation → pulmonary congestion→ pulmonary edema, pulmonary artery high

浮肿
- 二尖瓣关闭不全
  - 血流动力学 累及心脏收缩期
  - 二尖瓣关闭不全→部分血液反流左房→左房肥大扩张→左室肥大扩张→肺淤血、肺动脉高压→右室肥大扩张→右房肥大扩张→右心衰竭→大循环淤血
  - X线 由于左心房和左心室同时扩大呈球形心
  - 听诊 心尖区收缩期吹风样杂音
  - 症状 左心衰竭及右心衰竭
- 主动脉瓣狭窄
  - 血流动力学 累及心脏收缩期
  - 主动脉瓣狭窄→左室排血受阻→左室向心性肥大→失代偿扩张→左房肥大扩张→肺淤血肺动脉高压→右室肥大扩张→右房肥大扩张→大循环淤血,类似高血压心脏病

pressure→right ventricular hypertrophy and dilatation →right atrial hypertrophy and expansion→ right heart failure, like hypertensive hear disease

- ○ X-ray   Boot shaped heart
- ○ Auscultation   Systolic ejection murmur in aortic area
- ○ Signs   cardiac output decreased, Coronary artery perfusion reduce, Pulse pressure decreased, Syncope and sudden death

● Aortic insufficiency

- ○ Hemodynamic changes   involving diastolic phase
- ○ Aortic insufficiency→part blood reflux into left ventriculum → left ventricular hypertrophy and dilatation→ left atrial hypertrophy and dilatation → pulmonary congestion and pulmonary artery high pressure→right ventricular hypertrophy and dilatation, →right atrial hypertrophy and expansion → right heart failure
- ○ X-ray   Boot shaped heart
- ○ Auscultation   Aortic diastolic blowing murmur
- ○ Signs   the gap of systolic and diastolic BPH increased angina pectoris

- ○ X线   靴形心
- ○ 听诊   主动脉瓣区收缩期粗糙喷射性杂音
- ○ 症状   冠状动脉灌注不足，脉压差减小，晕厥猝死

● 主动脉瓣关闭不全

- ○ 血流动力学   累及心脏舒张期

- ○ 主动脉瓣关闭不全→主动脉内血液反流→左室肥大扩张→左房肥大扩张→右室、右房肥大扩张→大循环淤血

- ○ X线   靴形心
- ○ 听诊   主动脉瓣舒张期吹风样杂音
- ○ 症状   脉压差增大，心绞痛

Section 6　Cardiomyopathy

Conception

- Primary cardiomyopathy is a kind of myocardial diseases mainly associated with cardiac dysfunction without definite etiology

Types

- Dilated cardiomyopathy
  - Dilated cardiomyopathy is characterized by failure of ventricle to empty in systole
  - The ventricular end of systolic and diastolic volume are increased causing bilateral ventricular dilation and failure
  - Commonly occur in 20～50 years old male with signs and symptoms of heart failure and sudden death
  - Grossly　Heart weight increased, heart chambers expansion, heart apex become round, intimal thickening and mural thrombus formation
  - Microscopically　Myocardial hypertrophy and atrophy, degeneration, focal necrosis interstitial fibrosis
- Hypertrophic cardiomyopathy
  - Hypertrophic cardiomyopathy is

第6节　心肌病

概述

- 原发性心肌病是指一组不明原因的与心肌功能异常相关的心肌疾病

类型

- 扩张性心肌病
  - 扩张性心肌病是收缩期心室排空衰竭
  - 双侧心室衰竭扩张导致心室收缩期和舒张期体积增大
  - 常见于20～50岁男性，表现为心力衰竭和猝死
  - 大体　心脏重量增加，心脏扩大，心尖圆钝，心内膜增厚，附壁血栓
  - 镜下　心肌肥大，萎缩，变性，灶性坏死和纤维化
- 肥厚型心肌病
  - 肥厚型心肌病特征是心室明显肥

characterized by marked hypertrophy of the ventricular muscle with resistance to diastolic filing. Both ventricles are diffusely involved in most cases

○ Clinically Low cardiac output, Pulmonary hypertension, Embolism. About 50% familial factors

○ Grossly Cardiac enlargement, Both sides of ventricular wall were hypertrophy, Interventricular septal thickness, Papillary muscle hypertrophy

○ Microscopically Myocardial cell diffuse hypertrophy, the myocardial fibers arrange disorder

● Restrictive cardiomyopathy
○ Restrictive cardiomyopathy is characterized by ventricular diastolic volume reduced

○ Grossly Cardiac stenosis, Endocardial and subendocardial fibrous thickening, gray, up to 2 ～ 3 mm, much severe in cardiac apex

○ Microscopically Endocardial fibrosis, hyaline degeneration, calcification, subendocardial atrophy, degeneration and myocardial fibrosis

● Keshan disease
○ It is local endemic disease firstly found in Heilongjiang Keshan

大, 舒张期心室充盈受限所致, 大部分病例累及双侧心室

○ **临床表现** 心输出量低, 肺动脉高压, 栓塞, 大约50%的家庭遗传因素

○ **大体** 心脏扩大, 心室两侧均肥大, 室间隔增厚, 乳头肌肥大, 心室狭窄

○ **镜下** 心肌细胞弥漫性肥大, 心肌纤维排列紊乱

● **限制型心肌病**
○ 限制型心肌病特征是心室舒张容积减少

○ **大体** 心脏狭窄, 心内膜和心内膜下纤维增厚, 变灰, 厚2～3毫米, 心尖部尤为明显

○ **镜下** 心内膜纤维化, 透明变性、钙化, 心内膜下萎缩、变性和心肌纤维化

● **克山病**
○ 克山病是地方流行病, 最早发现于黑龙江克山县, 在山区和丘陵

County, which prevalent in the mountainous and hilly areas

○ **Cause** lack of selenium and other elements in soil

○ **Grossly** Heart enlarged, weight increase, chambers of the heart enlarged, ventricular wall become thinner with scar

○ **Microscopically** Myocardial hydropic degeneration, Fatty degeneration, coagulative myocytolysis, fibrosis with scar

地区流行

○ **原因** 土壤中缺乏硒和其他元素

○ **大体** 心脏扩大，重量增加，心脏扩大，心壁变薄，瘢痕形成

○ **镜下** 心肌水变性，脂肪变性，凝固性肌溶解，纤维化和瘢痕形成

Section 7 Myocarditis

第7节　心肌炎

● Viral myocarditis
  ○ **Virus** Coxsackie virus, influenza virus, the virus directly damaged myocardium
  ○ **Grossly** The heart volume is slightly increased
  ○ **Microscopically** Myocardial interstitial lymphocyte
  ○ **Clinically** Arrhythmia
● Bacterial myocarditis
  ○ Caused by bacterial infection
● Isolated myocarditis
  ○ Also called idiopathic myocarditis,
  ○ The reasons is unknown.
  ○ Type

● **病毒性心肌炎**
  ○ **病毒** 柯萨奇病毒，流感病毒等，病毒直接破坏心肌
  ○ **大体** 心脏略增大
  ○ **镜下** 心肌间质淋巴、单核细胞浸润
  ○ **临床** 心律失常
● **细菌性心肌炎**
  ○ 由细菌感染所致
● **孤立性心肌炎**
  ○ 又称特发性心肌炎
  ○ 原因不明
  ○ 类型

Diffuse interstitial myocarditis

Idiopathic giant cell myocarditis

- Immune myocarditis
  - Common in allergic diseases, rheumatism of heart
  - Microscopically Myocardial interstitial inflammation, Inflammatory cells infiltrated surrounding the small blood vessels in myocardial interstitial tissue with lymphocyte and histocytes

弥漫性间质性心肌炎

特发性巨细胞性心肌炎

- 免疫性心肌炎
  - 多见于变态反应性疾病、风湿性心脏病
  - 镜下　心肌间质炎，炎细胞位于心肌间质小血管周围，以淋巴细胞和组织细胞为主

朱光浩　何妙侠

Chapter 7

Diseases of Respiratory System

第7章

呼吸系统疾病

Section 1　Pneumonia

第1节　肺炎

🖋 Conception

- Acute pneumonia is an acute inflammation of the lung parenchyma resulting from infection of alveoli and respiratory bronchioles
- Acute pneumonia is characterized clinically by fever, cough, dyspnea, and chest-pain

🖋 概述

- 急性肺炎是感染引起的肺实质包括肺泡到呼吸性细支气管的急性炎症

- 临床上急性肺炎以发热、咳嗽、呼吸困难和胸痛为特征

🖋 Lobar pneumonia

Definition

- Lobar pneumonia is an acute inflammation caused by pneumococci with fibrous exudation in the alveoli
- It always involves lobar of the lung and absence of involvement of bronchi
- It is much more prevalent at the youngers
- Lower lobes or the right middle lobe

🖋 大叶性肺炎

定义

- 大叶性肺炎是肺炎球菌感染所引起的以肺泡内弥漫性纤维素渗出为主的一种急性炎症
- 累及肺大叶,不累及支气管

- 年轻人多见

- 以右肺中、下叶最常累及

is the most frequently involved

- Streptococcus pneumoniae is responsible for more than 90% of lobar pneumonias

Pathological features

- Lobar pneumonia progresses through four stages: congestion, red hepatization, gray hepatization and resolution

Stage 1   Congestion 1～2 days

- Grossly   The affected lobe of lung is heavy, boggy, and red
- Microscopically   It is characterized by vascular engorgement, intra-alveolar fluid with few neutrophils, and often the presence of numerous bacteria
- Clinically   X-ray showed large thin and uniform shadows. The patient is coughing up white foamy sputum

Stage 2   Red hepatization 3～4 days

- Grossly   the lobe is red, firm, and airless like liver
- Microscopically   It is characterized by massive confluent exudation, such as neutrophils, red cells, and fibrin fill the alveolar spaces
- Clinically   The patient has cyanosis, rusty sputum and X-ray shows dense shadow in lung lobe

Stage 3   Gray hepatization 5～6 days

- Grossly   The lung is resulting in a

- 肺炎链球菌感染占大叶性肺炎的90%以上

病理特征

- 大叶性肺炎分四期：充血水肿期，红色肝样变期，灰色肝样变期和溶解消散期

第1期   充血水肿期第1～2天

- 大体   受累肺叶增大，重量增加，暗红色
- 镜下   肺泡隔毛细血管扩张充血，肺泡腔内大量渗出液，伴少量中性粒细胞，常可检出细菌
- 临床上   X线显示大片淡薄均匀阴影，患者咳白色泡沫痰

第2期   红色肝样变期第3～4天

- 大体   肺叶增大，重量增加，暗红，质实无气如肝
- 镜下   以大量渗出，相互融合为特征，包括大量中性粒细胞、红细胞及纤维素充填于肺泡腔内
- 临床上   患者发绀，咳铁锈色痰，X线示肺叶大片致密阴影

第3期   灰色肝样变期第5～6天

- 大体   肺叶肿大，灰白色，质实

color change to grayish-brown like liver

○ Microscopically Capillaries in the wall of alveoli are compressed leads to hyperemia regressed. It is marked by progressive disintegration of red cells and the persistence of a fibrinosuppurative exudate

○ Clinically The patients have high fever, chest pain with mucous and purulent sputum without bacteria. Dyspnea and cyanosis lessened. X-ray shows dense shadow in the lung lobe.

Stage 4 Resolution 7 days (1w)

○ Grossly The affected lobe become soft and recovery

○ Microscopically The exudate within the alveolar spaces is broken down by enzymatic digestion to produce granular, semifluid debris that is resorbed, ingested by macrophages, expectorated, or organized by fibroblasts

○ Clinically The temperature of patients is normal and X-rays show the shade of lung lesion disappeared

Complications

● Pulmonary carnification Also called organized pneumonia. The

如肝

○ **镜下** 肺泡壁毛细血管受压，充血消退。突出表现为红细胞的渗出减少与大量脓性纤维素渗出之间的分离现象

○ **临床上** 患者高热，胸痛，咳黏液脓痰，不含细菌。呼吸困难和发绀减轻。X线显示肺叶致密阴影

第4期 溶解消散期第7天（1周）

○ **大体** 肺叶实变病灶消失，质地变软

○ **镜下** 肺泡腔内中性粒细胞坏死，释放蛋白水解酶溶解纤维素，被巨噬细胞吞噬或咳出，或被纤维母细胞机化

○ **临床上** X线示阴影逐渐消散，体温恢复正常

并发症

● **肺肉质变** 亦称机化性肺炎。由于中性粒细胞渗出较少，释放的蛋白水

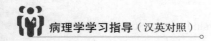

lesion areas of the lung organized and convert the intra-alveolar exudate to solid fibrous tissue because of fewer enzymatic resolution by neutrophils, looks like brown flesh

- Fibrinous or fibrinopurulent pleuritic Pleural fibrinous reaction to the underlying inflammation is often present in the early stages if the consolidation extends to the surface (pleuritis). It may resolve or undergo organization, leaving fibrous thickening or permanent adhesions

- Abscess The lung inflammation and necrosis may lead to abscess formation, sometimes with sepsis and infective shock

Lobular pneumonia (Bronchopneumonia)

Definition

- Lobular pneumonia is characterized by foci of acute suppurative inflammation centered on bronchioles

- In bronchopneumonia, the terminal bronchioles infected, with involvement of adjacent alveoli in a patchy

- It is much more prevalent at the elder of age or children, and patient staying in bed

- It is often caused by a variety of

解酶不足，纤维素溶解不完全，被肉芽组织取代机化，呈褐色肉样

- **胸膜肥厚和粘连** 发生纤维素性胸膜炎常出现在早期渗出后累及胸膜表面，纤维素吸收不完全而致胸膜粘连

- **脓肿** 肺组织损伤和坏死伴脓肿形成，有时伴败血症及感染性休克

小叶性肺炎（支气管肺炎）

定义

- 小叶性肺炎是以细支气管为中心的化脓性炎症

- 病变主要累及终末细支气管，周围肺组织呈斑片状受累

- 主要发生于儿童、体弱老人和久病卧床者

- 常由多种细菌引起，如葡萄球菌、肺

bacteria, such as staphylococcus, pneumococcus, etc.

Pathological features

- Grossly
  - Focal inflammatory lesion is distributed in patches throughout one or several lobes, most frequently involving bilateral and basal area of lung
  - The lesions up to 0.5 ～ 1 cm in diameter and gray-red to yellow in color
  - The focal lesions are easily confluent in severe cases, producing the appearance of like lobar lesions
- Microscopically
  - The bronchiolar mucosa is congested, edematous, and has mucous exudates on the mucosa surface
  - The bronchiolar lumen and surrounding alveolar spaces are filled with neutrophils and the exfoliated epithelium
  - The surrounding lung tissue is congested, and some alveoli have compensatory emphysema

Complications

- Abscess
- Empyema
- Bacterial dissemination meningitis, infective endocarditis, heart, and pulmonary function failure

炎球菌等

病理特征

- 大体
  - 肺一叶或多叶表面和切面散在分布病灶,常累及双侧肺,以基底段多见
  - 病变大小为0.5～1厘米,呈灰黄色
  - 病灶常常容易融合成片甚至形成像大叶性肺炎外观
- 镜下
  - 支气管黏膜淤血、水肿,黏膜表面有黏液性分泌物
  - 支气管腔及其周围肺泡见大量中性粒细胞及坏死碎屑
  - 周围肺组织淤血,部分肺泡代偿性肺气肿

并发症

- **肺脓肿**
- **肺气肿**
- **细菌感染播散** 肺炎性脑膜炎,感染性心内膜炎,心肺功能不全

Viral pneumonias

Definition

- Viral pneumonia mostly caused by influenza or parainfluenza viruses, also called interstitial pneumonia
- Microscopically   the alveolar septa are expanded by hyperemia, edema and inflammation cells infiltration composed of lymphocytes and plasma cells. Sometimes there are alveolar hyaline membrane formation
- Clinically   the patient present onset of fever, cough, and dyspnea. Cough usually unproductive or mucoid sputum
- The illness is usually mild and self-limited. Chest X-ray shows the pattern of interstitial involvement

Community-Acquired Acute Pneumonias

- It is infected follows a viral upper respiratory tract infection are secondary infection by bacteria
- It always shows interstitial pneumonia or with secondary suppurative inflammation
- Sometimes, the patients have abrupt onset of high fever, shaking chills, pleuritic chest pain, mucopurulent cough, and hemoptysis

Atypical Pneumonias

- The inflammation in the lungs is

病毒性肺炎

定义

- 病毒性肺炎大部分由流感病毒或副流感病毒引起，又称为间质性肺炎

- 镜下   病变肺泡隔增宽、充血、水肿伴淋巴细胞和浆细胞等炎症细胞浸润，有时肺泡形成透明膜

- 临床上   病人可以出现发热、咳嗽、呼吸困难。咳嗽无痰或黏液痰

- 也可表现轻微，或为自限性病程，胸部X线片示肺间质受累

社区获得性急性肺炎

- 常为上呼吸道病毒感染后继发细菌感染

- 表现为间质性肺炎或伴发继发性化脓性炎
- 有时可突发高热，发冷、胸膜炎性胸痛，黏液脓性咳嗽或咯血

非典型性肺炎

- 肺部炎症表现为斑片状，主要累及肺

focal patchy and largely confined to the alveolar septa and pulmonary interstitial septa

- Atypical refers to moderate volume of sputum, lack of typical presentation, moderate white blood cell count and lack of alveolar exudate
- Grossly the lesions are patchy, congested, and subcrepitant rale
- Microscopically the lesion is largely confined within the walls of the alveoli, alveoli septa are widened, edema and infiltrated by lymphocytes and plasma cells, the alveolar spaces are remarkably free of cellular exudate. Sometimes there are viral inclusion and multinucleated giant cells

Clinical Features

- Atypical pneumonia is extremely varied with different manifestation
- Coronavirus pneumonia 2019 is a kind of viral pneumonia endemic all over the world
- The patient has fever, headache, cough with minimal sputum
- It could be severe upper respiratory tract infection to fulminant, life-threatening infection in immunocompromised patients
- It can be used for auxiliary diagnosis

泡隔和肺间质

- 非典型是指痰量中等,缺乏典型表现,白细胞计数仅中度升高,肺泡缺乏渗出液
- **大体** 病变呈斑片状、淤血和有捻发音
- **镜下** 病变主要局限于肺泡隔,肺泡隔增宽、水肿伴淋巴、浆细胞浸润,肺泡腔无细胞渗出。有时可见病毒包涵体和多核巨细胞

临床特征

- 非典型肺炎临床表现变化大,常表现不同
- 新型冠状病毒感染属于全世界流行性病毒性肺炎
- 患者主要表现为发热、头痛、咳少量痰
- 免疫缺陷患者可出现严重的上呼吸道感染
- 可进行病毒、支原体抗原核酸检测等

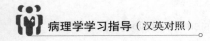

by virus, mycoplasma antigen nucleic acid detection

辅助诊断

Compare of three types of pneumonia

三种类型肺炎比较

Types	Lobar pneumonia	Lobular Pneumonia	Viral Pneumonia
Features	Fibrous inflammation	Bronchiole purulent inflammation	Alveoli septa inflammation
Causes	Pneumococcus	Multi bacteria	Virus Mycoplasma
Patients	Youth	Children Elder adults	Children
Location	Lobar	Lobular Confluent	Pulmonary interstitial area
Pathology	Four stages typical fibrous inflammation Alveolar structure free	Bronchiole purulent inflammation necrosis neutrophils	Alveoli septa Viral occlusion Multiple giant cells
Complications	Pulmonary cornification	Abscess Heart failure Sepsis	Hyaline membrane formation
Prognosis	Well	Poor	Well Can be cured

类型	大叶性肺炎	小叶性肺炎	病毒性肺炎
特征	纤维素性炎	细支气管为中心的化脓性炎	肺泡隔炎症
病因	肺炎球菌感染	多种细菌感染	病毒、支原体
发病人群	青壮年多见	小儿及年老者	儿童多见
部位	累及肺大叶	累及肺小叶亦可融合	肺间质
病理变化	四期变化典型过程肺泡结构保留	细支气管黏膜化脓性炎坏死中性粒细胞	肺泡隔增宽病毒包含体多核巨细胞
并发症	肺肉质变	脓肿、心衰、脓毒血症	透明膜形成
预后	预后好	预后不佳	预后好可痊愈

Acute Respiratory Distress Syndrome (ARDS)

急性呼吸窘迫综合征（ARDS）

Definition

- Acute Respiratory Distress Syndrome is clinical syndrome caused by diffuse

定义

- 急性呼吸窘迫综合征是由弥漫性肺泡毛细血管和上皮损害引起的临床

alveolar capillary and epithelial damage

Pathological feature

- Grossly   lungs are dark red, firm, airless, and heavy
- Microscopically   There are capillary congestion, necrosis of alveolar epithelial cells, interstitial and intra-alveolar edema, and hemorrhage, stasis of neutrophils in capillaries
- There are hyaline membrane formation lining the distended alveolar ducts, which is consist of fibrin-rich edema fluid admixed with necrotic epithelial cells and remarkably similar to that seen in respiratory distress syndrome in the newborn (NRDS)

Clinical features

- Rapid onset of life-threatening respiratory insufficiency, cyanosis, and severe arterial hypoxemia that is refractory to oxygen therapy and progress to multisystem and organ failure

Section 2   Chronic obstructive pulmonary disease (COPD)

Conception

- COPD is a group of disorders

综合征

病理特征

- **大体**   肺呈深红色,坚硬,无气且较重
- **镜下**   毛细血管充血,肺泡上皮细胞坏死,间质和肺泡内有水肿及出血,毛细血管中性粒细胞瘀滞

- 透明膜形成由富含纤维蛋白的水肿液与坏死上皮细胞的残留物混合而成,与新生儿呼吸窘迫综合征(NRDS)相似

临床特征

- 快速出现的危及生命的呼吸功能不全,发绀和严重的动脉供氧不足,进而发展为多系统器官衰竭

第2节   慢性阻塞性肺疾病(COPD)

概述

- COPD是一组以呼吸困难为主要表

characterized by dyspnea. There are four disorders in COPD: Chronic bronchitis, Emphysema, Bronchial asthma and Bronchiectasis

Chronic bronchitis

Definition

- Chronic bronchitis is a chronic nonspecific inflammatory disease occurring in bronchial mucosa and surrounding tissues

Diagnostic criteria

- There are persistent productive cough for at least 3 months in 2 years continuously

Etiology and pathogenesis

- Infection of bacteria and virus
- Smoking
- Pollution and allergy
- Lower immune function

Pathological changes

- Grossly
  - Larger airways usually hyperemic and covered with mucosal secretions
  - Secretions are mucinous or mucopurulent
  - Smaller bronchi and bronchioles filled with secretions in the late stage
- Microscopically
  - The goblet cells of epithelial cells

现的呼吸系统疾病,包括慢性支气管炎,支气管哮喘,肺气肿和支气管扩张

慢性支气管炎

定义

- 慢性支气管炎是发生在支气管黏膜及其周围组织的慢性非特异性炎症性疾病

诊断标准

- 反复发作的咳嗽、咳痰或伴有喘息症状,且症状每年持续3个月以上,连续发病2年以上

病因病机

- 细菌或病毒感染
- 吸烟
- 环境污染及过敏
- 机体免疫系统功能低下

病理变化

- 大体
  - 大气道充血,表面覆盖黏液性分泌物
  - 分泌物可以是黏液性或黏液脓性
  - 病变后期小气道及细支气管充满分泌物
- 镜下
  - 上皮细胞杯状细胞增多, 出现

increased, and squamous cells appeared

○ Gland hyperplasia and hypertrophy, more mucous glands than serous glands, secreting a lot of mucus

○ Smooth muscle rupture and atrophy, cartilage degeneration, atrophy, and ossification. The lumen is irregular

○ Congestion and edema of the vessel wall, infiltration of lymphocytes, plasma cells and a small amount of neutrophils

○ The lesions spread from the large bronchi to the small bronchi, the bronchiolar walls were fibrotic and thickened, and the lumen was narrowed

Clinical features

● In early stages of the disease, the productive cough raises mucoid sputum, and acute with mucopurulent, but airflow is not obstructed

● Some patients with chronic bronchitis may demonstrate hyperresponsive airways with intermittent bronchospasm and wheezing

● Some patients as heavy smokers have chronic outflow obstruction, usually develop emphysema

Consequences

● Recovered

鳞化

○ 腺体增生肥大,黏液腺多于浆液腺,分泌大量黏液

○ 平滑肌断裂和萎缩,软骨变性、萎缩、骨化。管腔不规则

○ 血管管壁充血水肿,淋巴细胞、浆细胞及少量中性粒细胞浸润

○ 病变从大支气管向小支气管蔓延,细支气管管壁纤维化增厚,管腔狭窄

临床特征

● 早期以咳白色黏液泡沫痰,急性发作时为黏液脓性痰,气道阻塞不明显

● 部分患者表现为气道高反应,伴有间歇性支气管痉挛和喘息

● 重度吸烟者的患者有慢性流出道梗阻,通常发展为肺气肿

结局

● 痊愈

- Acute attack with acute suppurative bronchitis
- Secondary emphysema, cor pulmonale, complicated with bronchiectasis

Bronchial asthma

Definition

- Bronchial asthma is short for asthma
- Chronic inflammatory disorder of the airways that causes recurrent episodes of wheezing, breathlessness, chest tightness, and cough, particularly at night and/or early in the morning

Etiology and pathogenesis

- There exist allergens
- Patient has an allergic possibility to environment substances

Pathological changes

- Grossly
  - The lungs are over distended because of overinflation
  - Occlusion of bronchi and bronchioles by thick, tenacious mucous plugs
- Microscopically
  - The mucus plugs contain whorls of shed epithelium (Curschmann spirals)
  - Numerous eosinophils and Charcot-Leyden crystals (collections of crystalloids made up of eosinophil proteins)

- 急性发作,常伴发急性化脓性支气管炎
- 继发肺气肿、肺心病;并发支气管扩张症

支气管哮喘

定义

- 简称哮喘
- 由呼吸道过敏引起的以支气管可逆性发作性痉挛为特征。表现为反复发作伴有哮鸣音的呼气性呼吸困难、咳嗽、胸闷等,尤其是夜间及早晨易发作

病因与病机

- 存在过敏原
- 某些患者易于对外界环境物质过敏

病理变化

- 大体
  - 肺因过度充气而膨胀
  - 支气管及细支气管伴厚而坚韧的黏液栓堵塞
- 镜下
  - 黏液栓中含脱落的上皮(库施曼螺旋体)
  - 较多嗜酸粒细胞及夏科–莱登晶体(嗜酸性蛋白构成的结晶体)

○ Airway remodeling, including

A Thickening of basement membrane of the bronchial epithelium

B Edema and inflammatory infiltrate in the bronchial walls with a prominence of eosinophil and mast cells

C Increase in the size of the submucosal glands

D Hypertrophy of muscles in the bronchial walls

Clinical-pathological features

- Bronchial constriction and mucus embolism leading to expiratory dyspnea and wheezing
- Complications
  ○ Chronic bronchitis
  ○ Bronchiectasis
  ○ Emphysema
  ○ Corpulmonale

Bronchiectasis

Definition

- Bronchiectasis is characterized with persistent dilatation of small and middle bronchus in the lung with fibrous thickening
- The patients always have chronic cough, a large amount of purulent sputum and repeated hemoptysis

○ 气道重建,包括

A 支气管上皮细胞基底膜增厚

B 支气管壁水肿伴炎症细胞浸润,以嗜酸性粒细胞、肥大细胞浸润最明显

C 支气管黏膜下腺体增大

D 支气管壁平滑肌肥大

临床病理特征

- 细支气管痉挛和黏液栓塞引起呼气性呼吸困难伴哮鸣音

- 并发症
  ○ 慢性支气管炎
  ○ 支气管扩张
  ○ 肺气肿
  ○ 肺心病

支气管扩张症

定义

- 支气管扩张是指肺内小支气管持久性扩张伴管壁纤维性增厚为特征的慢性呼吸道疾病

- 临床表现为慢性咳嗽,大量脓痰及反复咯血

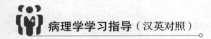

- Secondary from chronic bronchitis

Pathological changes

- Grossly
  - The airways dilated involving bilateral pulmonary lower lobes, maybe related to the pleural surfaces
  - The bronchus dilated as cylinders or cysts
  - There were minus purulent or yellowish-green purulent exudate in the bronchial lumen

- Microscopically
  - There an intense acute and chronic inflammatory exudate within the walls of the bronchi and bronchioles, and desquamation and ulceration of epithelium in acute cases
  - There were fibrosis in the bronchial and bronchiolar walls and atrophy in the peribronchiolar
  - Necrosis destroys the bronchial or bronchiolar walls, leading to the formation of an abscess cavity

Clinical-pathological features

- Severe, persistent cough with muco-purulent sputum, the sputum may contain flecks of blood
- Clubbing of the fingers
- Mixed flora can be cultured from sputum
- Complications: pulmonary abscess,

- 多继发于慢性支气管炎

病理变化

- 大体
  - 常累及双肺下叶气道扩张，甚至近胸膜
  - 支气管呈圆柱状或囊状扩张
  - 支气管腔内有黏液脓性或黄绿色脓性渗出物

- 镜下
  - 急性病例支气管黏膜脱落或溃疡形成、管壁多量炎性渗出，黏膜下淋巴细胞、浆细胞及中性粒细胞浸润
  - 支气管壁纤维化、周围肺组织萎缩
  - 支气管壁因坏死等破坏导致脓肿腔形成

临床病理特征

- 频繁咳嗽，咳出大量黏脓痰，也可咯血
- 杵状指
- 痰液培养成混合细菌
- 并发症：肺脓肿，脓气肿，脓胸，肺心

empyema, pyneumothorax, pulmonary heart disease, etc.

病等

Emphysema

肺气肿

Definition

定义

- Pulmonary emphysema is a common complication of bronchial and pulmonary diseases

- 肺气肿是支气管和肺部疾病的常见合并症

- because of hyperaeration of peripheral lung tissues accompanied by destruction of alveolar septum, resulting in decreased elasticity of lung tissues, lung volume enlargement and function declined

- 末梢肺组织因含气量过多伴肺泡隔破坏,肺组织弹性下降,导致肺体积膨大、功能下降

- The cause was obstructive ventilation disorder; decreased of respiratory bronchial and alveolar elasticity and α1-antitryptase levels

- 病因是阻塞性通气障碍；呼吸性支气管和肺泡弹性降低；α1-抗胰蛋白酶水平降低

Types

类型

Centrilobular (Centri-acinar) Emphysema

中央型肺气肿

- The main causes are respiratory bronchioles or cigarette smoking

- 主要原因是支气管扩张或吸烟

- Most patients do not have congenital deficiency of α1-antitrypsin

- 多数病人无先天性 α1-抗胰蛋白酶缺乏

- The central or proximal parts of the pulmonary acini are affected, while distal alveoli are spared

- 病变发生在肺泡近段或中央,远段肺泡不受累

- Enlargement of central acinus and respiratory bronchioles

- 腺泡中央型呼吸性支气管囊状扩张

Distal Acinar (Peri-acinar) Emphysema

周围型肺气肿

- The proximal portion of the acinus is normal but the distal part is primarily

- 病变发生在肺泡远端,肺泡近段不受影响

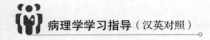

involved

- Along the lobular connective tissue septa and striking adjacent to the pleura
- Enlargement of peri-acinus and acinus
- Adjacent to areas of fibrosis, scarring, or atelectasis and is usually more severe in the upper half of the lungs
- Enlarged air spaces ranging in diameter from 0.5 mm to 2.0 cm, cystic structures progressive enlargement, are referred to as bullae

Pan-lobular (Pan-acinar) Emphysema

- The acini are completely enlarged, from the respiratory bronchiole to the terminal blind alveoli
- Pan-acinar emphysema tends to enlargement including respiratory bronchiole, alveolar ducts, and sacs
- It always involving the lower lobe of lung and because of $\alpha 1$-antitrypsin deficiency

Pathological changes

- Grossly
  - The lung looks pale, enlargement
  - It looks like honeycomb in cut surface of lung
- Microscopically
  - In addition to alveolar loss, the number of alveolar capillaries is diminished

- 腺泡周围型周围的肺泡管和肺泡囊扩张

- 常沿肺间质，并与胸膜相连
- 邻近纤维，瘢痕或支气管扩张者以肺上叶较严重

- 扩张直径0.5毫米至2厘米，甚至似桶状胸

全腺泡肺气肿

- 肺腺泡完全扩张，从呼气性细支气管到肺泡盲端

- 全腺泡型包括呼吸性支气管、肺泡管、肺泡囊、肺泡都扩张

- 肺下叶多发，与α1-抗胰蛋白酶缺乏有关

病理变化

- 大体
  - 肺苍白少血，体积增大
  - 切面呈蜂窝状

- 镜下
  - 肺泡数量减少，肺泡扩大，相互融合，毛细血管减少

- Terminal and respiratory bronchioles may be deformed because of the loss of septa
- With the loss of elastic tissue in the surrounding alveolar septa, radial traction on the small airways is reduced
- Chronic airflow obstruction
- Bronchiolar inflammation and submucosal fibrosis are consistently present in advanced disease

Clinical Features

- Dyspnea, Cough and wheezing, Weight loss
- Pulmonary function reduced, Barrel-chest, Chronic bronchitis and a history of recurrent infections with purulent sputum
- Secondary pulmonary hypertension

Section 3   Pneumoconiosis

Conception

- Pneumoconiosis consists of a group of chronic fibrotic diseases of the lung resulting from exposure to organic and inorganic particles, most commonly mineral dust
- Pulmonary alveolar macrophages play a central role in the pathogenesis

- 肺间隔变窄导致终末呼吸性细支气管变形
- 周围肺间隔弹性下降、收缩而导致小气道减少
- 慢性气道堵塞
- 晚期病变可有细支气管慢性炎和黏膜下纤维化

临床病理联系

- 呼吸困难,咳嗽和喘息,体重减轻
- 肺功能下降,桶状胸,慢性支气管炎,反复呼吸道感染
- 最终导致肺动脉高压

第3节   肺尘埃沉着病

概述

- 肺尘埃沉着病(又称尘肺病)是一组由于接触有机和无机颗粒(最常见的是矿物粉尘)而引起的慢性肺纤维化疾病
- 肺泡巨噬细胞在肺尘埃沉着病发病中起着关键的作用

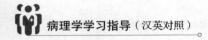

Silicosis

- Silicosis is the most common pneumoconiosis in the world, it is including the silicosis nodule formation and diffuse fibrosis
- The lesions showed asymptomatic silicosis nodules to progressive massive fibrosis, increased susceptibility to tuberculosis
- Microscopically, silicosis is characterized with hyaline nodule and diffuse fibrosis
- Silicosis nodule is clear nodule with a feeling of grittiness

Asbestosis

- Asbestosis is lung disease caused by long-term inhalation of asbestos fibers
- The lung shows diffuse fibrosis, pleural plaques, and thickening

Section 4　Tumors of respiratory system

Nasopharyngeal Carcinoma

- Nasopharyngeal carcinoma (NPC) is the common carcinoma from nasopharyngeal epithelial cells, mostly related to Epstein-Barr virus
- NPC is sensitive to chemotherapy, and chemotherapy combined with

矽肺

- 矽肺是世界范围内最常见的尘肺病，表现为矽结节的形成和肺纤维化
- 病变表现为无症状性矽结节形成到进行性纤维化，且容易感染结核
- 镜下，矽肺以透明变结节和弥漫性纤维化为特征
- 矽结节是具有砂砾感的透明结节

石棉肺

- 石棉肺是长期吸入石棉纤维导致的肺疾病
- 表现为肺弥漫性纤维化、胸膜增厚和胸膜斑块形成

第4节　呼吸系统肿瘤

鼻咽癌

- 鼻咽癌是来源于鼻咽上皮的常见恶性肿瘤，多数与EB病毒密切相关
- 鼻咽癌对化疗、放疗联合化疗敏感

radiotherapy

- Grossly, mucous membrane roughness or slightly elevated, or the formation of small nodules

- Microscopically, it can be divided into carcinoma in situ and invasive carcinoma, the later dominated by squamous carcinoma

Carcinoma of the lung

Conception

- Smoking is the most important risk factor of lung cancer

- Lung cancer classified as small cell carcinoma (SCLC) and non-small cell carcinoma (NSCLC)

- Adenocarcinomas are the most common cancers overall and are especially common in women of nonsmokers

Pathological features

- Three major histologic subtypes of lung cancer are adenocarcinoma (most common), squamous cell carcinoma, and small cell carcinoma, each of which is clinically and genetically different

- Precursor lesions of lung cancer are including atypical adenomatous hyperplasia and adenocarcinoma in situ for adenocarcinomas, squamous dysplasia for squamous carcinoma

- 大体早期表现为黏膜粗糙或略隆起,或形成小结节

- 镜下分原位癌和浸润性癌,后者以鳞状细胞癌为主

肺癌

概述

- 吸烟是肺癌的危险因素

- 肺癌分小细胞肺癌和非小细胞肺癌

- 腺癌是最常见的肺癌,尤其多见于女性非吸烟人群

病理特征

- 肺癌主要包括三种组织学亚型:腺癌(最常见),鳞状细胞癌和小细胞癌,它们在病理形态、临床表现和遗传特征上均不同

- 癌前病变包括腺癌的非典型腺瘤性增生和原位腺癌以及鳞状癌的鳞状不典型增生

- Adenocarcinoma in situ is imply the tumor size is less than 3 cm in diameter characterized by growth along with pulmonary alveoli without stromal invasion

Clinical feature

- Lung cancers commonly cause a variety of paraneoplastic syndromes. SCLCs are best treated with chemotherapy. The other carcinomas may be curable by surgery if limited to the lung

- Targeted therapies of lung cancer, such as EGFR inhibitor therapy for adenocarcinomas with EGFR mutations (exon 18 to 21), can be effective, is an excellent example of personalized cancer therapy

- 原位腺癌是指直径＜3厘米,沿肺泡壁贴壁生长,没有间质浸润的肿瘤

临床特征

- 肺癌通常引起多种副肿瘤综合征。小细胞肺癌用化疗治疗效果好。其他肺癌如果局限于肺部,主要通过手术切除,可达到治愈

- 肺癌靶向治疗,针对具有*EGFR*基因突变(18～21号外显子)的腺癌的EGFR抑制剂治疗,效果肯定,是肿瘤个体化靶向治疗的较为成功的例子

朱光浩　何妙侠

Chapter 8

Diseases of Digestive System

第8章

消化系统疾病

Section 1　Gastritis

第1节　胃炎

🌿 Conception

- Gastritis is an inflammatory lesion of the gastric mucosa
- Gastritis can be divided into acute gastritis and chronic gastritis

🌿 概念

- 胃炎是胃黏膜的炎性病变

- 可分为急性胃炎和慢性胃炎

🌿 Acute Gastritis

Etiology and Pathogenesis

- The basic cause of acute gastritis is damage of the gastric epithelium
- Etiologic agents are the followings
  ○ Drugs
  ○ Toxic chemicals
  ○ Stress
  ○ Chemotherapy
  ○ Ischemia

Types

- Acute irritated gastritis
- Acute hemorrhagic gastritis

🌿 急性胃炎

病因和发病机制

- 急性胃炎的根本原因是胃黏膜上皮的受损
- 损伤因子包括
  ○ 药物
  ○ 有毒化学物
  ○ 压力
  ○ 化疗
  ○ 缺血

类型

- 急性刺激性胃炎
- 急性出血性胃炎

- Acute infective gastritis

Pathological Features

- Diffuse hyperemia of the mucosa
- Multiple small, superficial erosions
- Sometimes ulcers
- Variable necrosis of superficial glands
- Hemorrhage in the lamina propria

Clinical Features

- Mild dyspepsia
- Upper abdominal pain
- Nausea and vomiting

Chronic Gastritis

Conception

- Chronic gastritis is a chronic non-specific inflammation of gastric mucosa with a high incidence
- Chronic gastritis are classified as chronic non-atrophic gastritis, also called chronic superficial gastritis; and chronic atrophic gastritis

Chronic non-atrophic gastritis

- Pyloric atrium is the most common part involved

Pathological changes

- **Grossly** the mucosa hyperemia and edema with slight red in color; hemorrhage and erosion
- **Microscopically** infiltrate of lymphocytes and plasma cells, typically present within the lamina propria, often

- 急性感染性胃炎

病理特征

- 黏膜弥漫性充血
- 多个小而浅表的糜烂
- 有时形成溃疡
- 浅表腺体不同程度坏死
- 固有层可有出血

临床特征

- 轻度消化不良
- 上腹部疼痛
- 恶心、呕吐

慢性胃炎

概念

- 慢性胃炎是胃黏膜的慢性非特异性炎症，发病率高

- 慢性胃炎可分为慢性非萎缩性胃炎，又叫慢性浅表性胃炎；与慢性萎缩性胃炎

慢性非萎缩性胃炎

- 胃窦是最常见的病变部位

病理改变

- **大体** 黏膜充血、水肿、轻度变红，出血或糜烂

- **显微镜下** 可见淋巴细胞和浆细胞浸润；主要在固有层浸润，通常仅限于胃黏膜的上 1/3

limited to the upper third of the gastric mucosa

Clinical features

- Mostly recovery by treatment or healthy diets
- Seldom transfer to chronic atrophic gastritis

Chronic atrophic gastritis

Types

- Type A   which is an autoimmune gastritis that primarily involves the fundus and body of stomach and is associated with pernicious anemia
- Type B   which primarily involves the antrum and is associated with Helicobacter pylori infection

Etiology

- H. Pylori: Helicobacter pylori (H. Pylori) is associated with numerous disease
- Chronic duodenal ulcer (100%)
- Chronic gastric ulcer (75%)
- Gastric adenocarcinoma (>80%)
- Malignant lymphoma (>60%)

Pathological changes

- Grossly
  - The color of mucosa changes from orange to gray
  - The layer of mucosa become thinner and looks like flattening

临床特征

- 大多经治疗或合理饮食而痊愈
- 少数转为慢性萎缩性胃炎

慢性萎缩性胃炎

类型

- A型   是一种自身免疫性胃炎，主要累及胃体和胃底，并伴有恶性贫血
- B型   主要累及胃窦并与幽门螺杆菌感染有关

病因学

- 幽门螺杆菌与多种疾病有关
- 慢性十二指肠溃疡（100%）
- 慢性胃溃疡（75%）
- 胃腺癌（>80%）
- 恶性淋巴瘤（>60%）

病理变化

- 大体
  - 黏膜颜色由橘红色变成灰色
  - 黏膜层变薄，皱襞变平整

- ○ The submucosal vessels are clearly visible
- Microscopically
  - ○ Mucosa layer become thinner, glands decreased in size and number
  - ○ Infiltrate of lymphocytes and plasma cells, maybe forming follicle
  - ○ Intestinal metaplasia
  - ○ Interstitial fibrosis

Clinical features

- Mild or severe dyspepsia
- Upper abdominal discomfort
- Rarely associated with carcinoma

Section 2　Peptic ulcer

Conception

- Peptic ulcer is chronic, most often solitary lesions that occur at any level of the GI tract that is exposed to the aggressive action of acid-peptic juices
- Two major subsets are gastric and duodenal
- They have different pathogenesis but similar morphology
- Duodenal ulcers are more likely than gastric ulcers

Epidemiology

- Peptic ulcers occur at all age, the most

- ○ 黏膜下血管清晰可见
- 镜下
  - ○ 黏膜变薄，黏膜腺体变小和数量减少
  - ○ 固有层淋巴、浆细胞浸润，有时可见淋巴滤泡
  - ○ 肠上皮化生
  - ○ 间质纤维组织增生

临床表现

- 轻度或严重消化不良
- 上腹部不适
- 极少数可癌变

第2节　消化性溃疡

概述

- 消化性溃疡是慢性常见单发性病变，可发生在胃肠道任何暴露于酸性消化液侵蚀的部位
- 胃和十二指肠是最常见的两个好发部位
- 其发病机制不同，但形态相似
- 十二指肠溃疡比胃溃疡更多见

流行病学

- 消化性溃疡可发生于任何年龄，主要

common age at onset is 20～40 years

- Male to female ratio = 3 : 1
- The familial tendency exists for duodenal ulcers but not for gastric ulcers
- Patients often have recurrent, periodic regularly upper abdominal pain

Pathogenesis

- Helicobacter pylori (HP) infection
  - H. pylori infection of the pyloric antrum is present in nearly all patients
  - Bacterial virulence factors such as the cytotoxin-associated gene pathogenicity island-encoded protein CagA and the vacuolating cytotoxin VacA aid in this colonization of the gastric mucosa and subsequently seem to modulate the host's immune system
- Gastric mucosal resistance impaired
  - Gastric mucosal secretion is decreased
  - The mucosa is injury
- Gastric acid digestion
  - Increased parietal cell in the stomach and hence a tendency to secrete more acid and pepsin
  - No acid, no ulcer
  - Abnormally rapid gastric emptying, exposing the duodenum to a greater

发生于 20～40 岁

- 男女之比 3 : 1
- 十二指肠溃疡存在家族倾向,而胃溃疡无

- 患者常有周期性规律性反复发作性上腹部疼痛

病因病机

- 幽门螺杆菌(HP)感染
  - 几乎所有病人都有胃窦部幽门螺杆菌感染
  - HP 感染可以释放细菌毒素因子如 CagA 和 VacA 于胃黏膜导致宿主免疫能力下降

- 黏膜抗消化能力降低
  - 胃黏膜黏液分泌减少

  - 黏膜受损
- 胃酸的消化作用
  - 胃壁细胞增多导致胃酸及胃蛋白酶分泌增多

  - 无酸无溃疡
  - 胃排空快导致十二指肠酸负荷增大

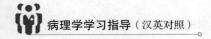

acid load

- Others
  - Stress, anxiety, and fatigue are associated with duodenal ulcers, especially with relapse, but the role of a "type A" personality is not proved
  - Use unbuffered aspirin, corticosteroids

🔖 Pathological Feature

- Grossly
  - 80% peptic ulcer are solitary lesions, with coexistence of gastric and duodenal ulcers in 10% ~ 20%
  - Classic peptic ulcer is a round-to-oval, sharply punched-out defect with relatively straight walls and essentially flat adjacent mucosa
  - Gastric ulcer primarily along the lesser curvature, mainly in the antrum, the posterior wall near the lesser curvature
  - Typically small, but size does not help differentiate between cancerous and benign gastric ulcers
  - Duodenal ulcer primarily in the first portion of the duodenum within a few centimeters of the pylorus, more often in the anterior

- 其他
  - 紧张、焦虑、疲劳与十二指肠溃疡有关，A 型性格是否与溃疡有关尚未证实

  - 口服无糖衣阿司匹林，可的松等药物

🔖 病理特征

- 大体
  - 80% 消化性溃疡为单发性病变，胃和十二指肠溃疡并存的比例为 10% ~ 20%

  - 典型的消化性溃疡是圆形到卵形的，边缘耸直，状如刀切，黏膜平坦

  - 胃溃疡主要沿胃小弯，累及胃窦，后壁靠近胃小弯

  - 通常小，但大小无助于区分胃癌和良性胃溃疡

  - 十二指肠溃疡主要在十二指肠的第一部分（球部），在幽门几厘米之内，多见于十二指肠前壁和后壁

wall and posterior wall

- Microscopically

  There are four layers of the ulcer base:

  ○ Zone 1　Active inflammation with neutrophils
  ○ Zone 2　Superficial layer of necrotic debris
  ○ Zone 3　Active granulation tissue
  ○ Zone 4　A base of scar tissue

  Surrounding wall

  ○ Mixed inflammation of mucosa (including eosinophils)
  ○ Blood vessels thickened, gastric or duodenal arteries and nerves may be eroded
  ○ Much scar tissues

Clinical features

- The patients always have recurrent intermittent regular upper abdominal pain
- Gastric ulcers show after meal pain which begin approximately 30 minutes after a meal, and is not relieved by eating
- Duodenal ulcers with hungry pain appear approximately 90 minutes after a meal, relieved by milk, food, antacids, vomiting

- 镜下

  溃疡底部有4层结构,由浅至深为:

  ○ 1层　以中性粒细胞为主的炎症区
  ○ 2层　表层坏死碎片区

  ○ 3层　肉芽组织为主
  ○ 4层　瘢痕组织层

  周边组织

  ○ 黏膜混合性炎症(包括嗜酸性粒细胞)
  ○ 增粗的血管,胃或十二指肠动脉、神经可能被侵蚀

  ○ 广泛的瘢痕组织

临床特征

- 患者常表现为反复发作的周期性间歇性上腹部疼痛

- 胃溃疡表现为饭后痛,饭后约30分钟就开始疼痛,进食并不会缓解疼痛,反而引起疼痛

- 十二指肠溃疡表现为饥饿痛,饭后约90分钟疼痛,进食牛奶、食物、抗酸剂,呕吐缓解

Complications

- Bleeding
  - Erosion of small artery in the base of a gastric ulcer causes bleed, which may be massive or occult repeated small hemorrhages
  - patient has hematemesis and hematochezia, subsequently anemia
- Pyloric obstruction
  - Stenosis from edema or scarring
- Perforation
  - The ulcerating process may extend deep into the muscular layer and even leads perforate led substance from stomach into the peritoneal cavity causing shock and peritonitis
  - Slow penetration results in a fibrous reaction
- Malignancy change
  - Malignancy do not occur in duodenal ulcers
  - Gastric ulcer may develop to carcinoma

Section 3   Appendicitis

Conception

- Appendicitis is the most common diseases of digestive system characterized by right lower quadrant pain and neutrophilic

并发症

- 出血
  - 胃溃疡基部的小动脉糜烂会导致出血，可能是大量出血或隐匿性反复小出血
  - 患者可有呕血和便血，进而导致贫血
- 幽门梗阻
  - 水肿或瘢痕引起的狭窄
- 穿孔
  - 溃疡过程可能延伸到肌肉层深处，甚至直接穿过壁，穿透到腹膜腔，引起休克和腹膜炎
  - 慢性穿孔常导致纤维反应
- 癌变
  - 十二指肠溃疡不会发生恶性肿瘤
  - 胃溃疡可发生癌变

第3节   阑尾炎

概念

- 阑尾炎是消化系统常见病，以右下腹疼痛和中性粒细胞升高为特征

leukocytosis

- Appendicitis can be divided into acute and chronic ones

Etiology

- Obstruction of the appendiceal lumen by a fecalith
- Colonic bacterial infection, mostly multiple bacteria's infection

Types

- Acute simple appendicitis
  - It is early appendicitis
  - Grossly   the appendix slightly edema and hyperemia on the surface of serosa
  - Macroscopically   there are inflammation involving mucosa and submucosa characterized by infiltrated by neutrophils
- Acute phlegmonous appendicitis
  - It is also called acute suppurative appendicitis
  - Grossly   the appendix severely edema, hyperemia and purulent exudation on the surface of serosa
  - Macroscopically   there are inflammation involving whole wall of appendix characterized by infiltrated by much of neutrophils

- 阑尾炎分急性和慢性

病因

- 阑尾腔粪石堵塞

- 肠道细菌感染,常为多种细菌感染

类型

- 急性单纯性阑尾炎
  - 阑尾早期炎症
  - 大体   阑尾轻度水肿和浆膜充血

  - 镜下   炎症主要累及黏膜及黏膜下层,以中性粒细胞浸润为特征

- 急性蜂窝织炎性阑尾炎
  - 又称急性化脓性阑尾炎

  - 大体   阑尾显著肿胀,浆膜面高度充血,表面可见脓苔

  - 镜下   炎症累及阑尾壁全层,以大量中性粒细胞浸润为特征

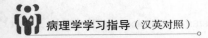

- Acute gangrenous appendicitis: Necrosis and perforation
  - Grossly the was necrosis and perforation in appendix wall with black or deep red in color
  - Microscopically there was necrosis of appendix wall and peritoneal suppurative inflammation

Clinical manifestation

- Fever, vomiting
- Peripheral blood shows neutrophilic leukocytosis
- Abdominal pain characterized by metastatic right lower quadrant pain

Complications

- Local extension of the inflammatory may involve the peri-appendiceal tissues and result in an inflammatory mass or abscess
- Appendix perforation into the peritoneal cavity may result in acute peritonitis

Section 4   Idiopathic inflammatory bowel disease (IBD)

Conception

- The term idiopathic inflammatory

- 急性坏疽性阑尾炎：坏死和穿孔
  - **大体** 阑尾壁坏死伴穿孔，色暗红或黑色
  - **镜下** 阑尾壁坏死，伴化脓性腹膜炎

临床表现

- 发热，呕吐
- 外周血白细胞升高
- 转移性右下腹疼痛

并发症

- 阑尾炎症扩展累及周围组织形成脓肿
- 阑尾穿孔引起急性腹膜炎

第4节   炎症性肠病

概念

- 炎症性肠病（IBD）一词用于克罗恩

bowel disease (IBD) is used for two diseases Crohn's disease and ulcerative colitis

- Although its cause is still not clear, the disease probably has an immunologic hypersensitivity basis
- They are recognized as distinct entities with distinct clinical and pathological features

Crohn's Disease

Etiology

- Crohn's disease occurs common in Western country
- Both sexes are affected equally
- It occurs at any age but has its highest incidence in young adults
- The cause of Crohn's disease is unknown
- Patients with active Crohn's disease frequently have T cell dysfunction

Pathological changes

- Location
  ○ The most common sites are terminal ileum, and colon
  ○ There has potential to involve any part of gastrointestinal tract from the mouths to the anus
- Grossly
  ○ It is characterized by involvement of discontinuous segments of

病和溃疡性结肠炎两种疾病

- 虽然病因尚不清楚,但该类疾病可能有超敏反应基础

- 克罗恩病和溃疡性结肠炎是具有不同临床和病理特征的不同实体

克罗恩病

病因

- 克罗恩病在西方国家多见

- 男女均可发病
- 可发生于任何年龄,但主要见于年轻人
- 病因不明

- 活动期常伴T细胞功能异常

病理变化

- 位置
  ○ 主要累及末端回肠及结肠

  ○ 病变可累及从口腔到肛门的胃肠道任何一个部位

- 大体
  ○ 病变肠管呈节段性改变(跳跃性病变)

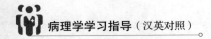

intestine (Skip lesions)

- ○ The affected segment is greatly thickened and rigid

- ○ Normal and affected intestine are sharply demarcated from one another

- ○ The affected part swollen and reddened, diffuse hyperemia, shallow ulceration, and thickness of whole intestinal wall

- ○ Fibrosis causes luminal narrowing with intestinal obstruction

- Microscopically

  - ○ Crohn's disease is characterized by distortion of mucosal crypt architecture, transmural inflammation, and slit ulceration

  - ○ The epithelioid granulomas are present with no caseous necrosis

  - ○ Fissures and fistulas of affected intestine may be present with marked fibrosis

  - ○ The regional mesenteric lymph nodes enlarged and may contain noncaseating granulomas

Clinical manifestation

- Chronic disease is characterized by remissions and relapses over a long period of time and may extremely be variable in clinical manifestation

- In the acute phase, patients present

- ○ 病变肠段增厚、僵硬

- ○ 病变肠段与正常肠段间隔呈节段状分界清楚

- ○ 黏膜肿胀,发红,浅表溃疡形成和管壁增厚

- ○ 病变肠段纤维化,肠腔狭窄,致肠梗阻

- 镜下

  - ○ 克罗恩病特征性表现是黏膜隐窝扭曲,穿壁性炎症和裂隙状溃疡

  - ○ 上皮样细胞肉芽肿,无干酪样坏死

  - ○ 可出现窦道及瘘管及明显纤维化

  - ○ 肠系膜淋巴结肿大,可见非干酪样坏死性肉芽肿

临床表现

- 克罗恩病临床表现变化大,呈慢性疾病特点,发作后很长一段时间才能缓解

- 急性期患者表现为发热、腹泻和右下

fever, diarrhea, and right lower quadrant pain mimic acute appendicitis

- Diagnosis is based on a combination of clinical, radiologic, and pathologic findings
- Chronic disease may be complicated by intestinal obstruction, fissures, and fistulas

Ulcerative Colitis
Etiology

- It is a colonic inflammatory disease of unknown cause
- It has a chronic course characterized by remissions and relapses
- It occurs commonly in the 20 to 30 years old age group, but may occur at any age
- Slightly females＞males

Pathological changes

- Location
  - Rectum, the disease extends proximally colon from the rectum
  - The lesions are in a continuous manner without skip areas
  - The mucosa has multiple erosions and shadow ulceration
- Grossly
  - The rough, red appearance of mucosa is characteristic but not specific

象限疼痛,类似急性阑尾炎

- 诊断基于临床、放射学和病理等综合分析

- 克罗恩病可并发肠梗阻、窦道及瘘管

溃疡性结肠炎
病因

- 病因不明的结肠炎性疾病

- 发作期与缓解期反复交替

- 任何年龄均可发病,以20～30岁多见

- 女性略多于男性

病理变化

- 位置
  - 主要累及直肠以及直肠附近的结肠
  - 病变连续无跳跃

  - 肠黏膜多发性糜烂或表浅溃疡

- 大体
  - 黏膜粗糙、发红但无特征性

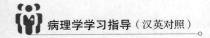
○ The mucosa diffusely hyperemia with superficial ulceration

○ The mucosa of around lesion polypoid proliferation

- Microscopically
  ○ The lesion mainly involves the superficial mucosa, the inflammation is usually restricted to the mucosa and submucosa
  ○ There was diffuse hyperemia with numerous superficial ulcerations in the acute phase
  ○ The mucosa crypt decreased and distortion, there were chronic inflammation cells infiltration in laminal propria and crypt abscess
  ○ There has polypoid proliferation leading pseudo-polyp formation

Clinical features

- In the acute phase and onset, the patient has fever, leukocytosis, lower abdominal pain, and diarrhea with blood and mucus in the stool

- Increased risk of developing colon carcinoma, about 10%

Section 5　Viral hepatitis

🖋 **Etiology and pathogenesis**

- Viral hepatitis is the common infectious

○ 黏膜弥漫性充血伴浅表溃疡形成

○ 周边黏膜息肉样增生

- 镜下
  ○ 病变主要位于浅表黏膜,病变局限于黏膜及黏膜下层

  ○ 急性期黏膜弥漫性充血伴多个浅表溃疡

  ○ 慢性期隐窝减少,变形,固有层较多慢性炎细胞浸润及隐窝脓肿

  ○ 病变周边黏膜息肉样增生伴假息肉形成

临床特征

- 急性期及发作期患者可有发热、白细胞增高,下腹疼痛,腹泻,大便带血和黏液

- 10%溃疡性结肠炎有发展为肠癌的风险

第5节　病毒性肝炎

🖋 **发病原因**

- 病毒性肝炎是一组肝炎病毒引起的

disease caused by a group of hepatitis virus leading hepatocyte degeneration and necrosis

- Common viruses: HAV, HBV, HCV, HDV, HEV, HFV

Basic pathological changes

- Liver cell degeneration
  - Ballooning degeneration
  - Acidophilic change
  - Fatty changes
- Liver cell necrosis
  - Spotty necrosis
  - Focal necrosis
  - Piecemeal necrosis
  - Bridging necrosis
  - Sub-massive/massive necrosis
- Inflammatory cells infiltration
  - Mainly infiltration by lymphocyte and monocyte in portal area and necrosis
- Regeneration
  - Hepatocytes regeneration
  - Stroma reactive proliferations
  - Ito cell hyperplasia, fibroblast proliferations

Etiology

- Viral hepatitis accounts for 50% ~ 65% of cases
- It may also result from drugs, poisoning

肝细胞变性、坏死为主要病变特征的常见传染病

- 常见的病毒包括HAV，HBV，HCV，HDV，HEV，HFV

基本病变

- 肝细胞变性
  - 气球样变
  - 嗜酸性变
  - 脂肪变性
- 肝细胞坏死
  - 点状坏死
  - 灶性坏死
  - 碎片状坏死
  - 桥接坏死
  - 亚大块/大块坏死
- 炎细胞浸润
  - 门管区和坏死区淋巴细胞和单核细胞浸润
- 再生
  - 肝细胞再生
  - 基质反应性增生
  - 贮脂细胞增生，成纤维细胞增生

病因学

- 病毒性肝炎占病例的50% ~ 65%
- 部分可能是由于药物，中毒

- Ischemia and hyperthermia (heat stroke)
- Autoimmune hepatitis, and reactivation of chronic HBV with or without HDV

Prognosis

- Hepatitis caused by HAV has well prognosis. About 5% ～ 10% HBV and 50% HCV infection hepatitis develop into chronic hepatitis
- About 1% or less of cases of acute hepatitis run a fulminant course with sub-massive or massive liver necrosis

Clinical pathological types

- Ordinary viral hepatitis
- Fulminant viral hepatitis

Ordinary viral hepatitis

- Acute Ordinary hepatitis
  - Grossly　The liver is slightly enlarged and more or less green, depending on the degree of hepatocellular damage and jaundice
  - Microscopically　The liver cells show cellular swelling and ballooning degeneration, spotted necrosis and eosinophilic body, and inflammatory cell in portal area
  - Clinically　The patient presented with pain in the liver area, elevated serum alanine aminotransferase

- 局部缺血和热射病（中暑）
- 自身免疫性肝炎以及伴有或不伴有HDV的慢性HBV的再激活引起的

预后

- HAV预后好。5%～10%的HBV和50%的HCV感染肝炎演变成慢性肝炎

- 大约1%或更少的急性肝炎病例会出现暴发性病程，并伴有亚大规模或大规模肝坏死

临床病理类型

- 普通型肝炎
- 急性重型肝炎

普通型肝炎

- 急性普通型肝炎
  - 大体　肝脏略微肿大，或多或少呈绿色，这取决于肝细胞损伤和黄疸的程度

  - 镜下　肝细胞水变性，气球样变。肝细胞可有点状坏死与嗜酸性小体，门管区少量炎细胞浸润

  - 临床上　病人出现肝区疼痛，血清谷丙转氨酶（SGPT）升高和肝功能异常

(SGPT), and abnormal liver function

- Chronic Ordinary hepatitis
  - Chronic hepatitis is defined as biochemical or serologic evidence of continuing inflammatory hepatic disease for more than 6 months
  - With symptoms and without steady improvement

- 慢性普通型肝炎
  - 慢性肝炎指持续性炎症性肝病超过6个月

  - 有症状且无持续改善的生化或血清学证据

Scheuer Classification for Chronic hepatitis

Activity of inflammation			Degree of fibrosis	
Grade	Portal area	Liver lobular	Stage	Significance
G0	No or slight	No	S0	No
G1	Inflammation	Inflammation, no necrosis	S1	Portal area enlarged (fibrosis)
G2	Mild Piecemeal necrosis	Spotted and focal necrosis, Acidophilic body	S2	Portal area fibrosis, normal Liver lobular structure
G3	Medium Piecemeal necrosis	Severe focal necrosis	S3	Portal area fibrosis and abnormal Liver lobular structure, no liver cirrhosis
G4	Severe Piecemeal necrosis	Bridge necrosis (Multi lobular)	S4	Maybe or definite liver cirrhosis

慢性肝炎分类（Scheuer 方案）

炎症活动度			纤维化程度	
分级	门管区周围	小叶内	分期	意义
G0	无或轻度炎症	无炎症	S0	无
G1	门管区炎症	有炎症，无坏死	S1	门管区扩大（纤维化）
G2	轻度碎片状坏死	点状、灶性坏死，或嗜酸性小体	S2	门管区周围纤维化，小叶周围保留
G3	中度碎片状坏死	重度灶性坏死	S3	纤维化伴小叶结构紊乱，无肝硬化
G4	重度碎片状坏死	桥接坏死（多小叶坏死）	S4	可能或肯定的肝硬化

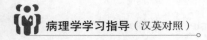

Fulminant Hepatitis

- Fulminant Hepatitis is defined as hepatic insufficiency progressing from onset to death (or hepatic transplantation) within 2 to 3 weeks
- The liver decreased in volume and microscopically shows massive necrosis
- A less rapid course extending up to 3 months is termed sub-massive necrosis

Section 6 Cholecystitis and pancreatitis

Cholecystitis and cholelithiasis

- Cholecystitis is caused by bacterial infection
- cholestasis is the basic lesion
- Always have cholelithiasis

Pancreatitis

- Acute pancreatitis tends to occur in middle-aged male after overeating or biliary tract disease
  - Acute edematous pancreatitis common in pancreatic tail, interstitial edema, neutrophils, monocytes infiltration, local necrosis
  - Acute hemorrhagic pancreatitis acute onset, severe, extensive bleeding necrosis, scattered in the calcium

急性重型肝炎

- 急性重型肝炎指2～3周内从发病到死亡（或肝移植）的肝功能不全

- 肝脏体积明显缩小,镜下显示大面积坏死
- 持续时间不超过3个月的较慢过程称为亚大块坏死

第6节 胆囊炎和胰腺炎

胆囊炎和胆石症

- 胆囊炎常由细菌感染引起

- 胆汁淤积是发病基础
- 常合并胆囊结石

胰腺炎

- **急性胰腺炎** 好发于中年男性暴饮暴食或胆道疾病后

  - **急性水肿性胰腺炎** 多见,胰腺尾部,间质水肿,中性粒细胞、单核细胞浸润,局部坏死

  - **急性出血胰腺炎** 发病急,病情重,广泛出血坏死,散在钙灶

focus

○ Clinical manifestations shock, peritonitis, increased hematuria amylase, decreased blood calcium, potassium, sodium

● Chronic pancreatitis partly related to autoimmune, with elevated serum IgG4

○ 临床表现 休克, 腹膜炎, 血尿淀粉酶升高, 血钙、钾、钠离子降低

● 慢性胰腺炎 部分与自身免疫有关, 血清 IgG4 水平升高

Section 7　Liver cirrhosis

🍃 Definition

Cirrhosis of the liver is a pathologic entity characterized by following Items

● Necrosis of liver cells, slowly progressive over a long period and ultimately causing chronic liver failure and death

● Fibrosis, which involves both liver lobular around central veins and portal areas

● Regenerative nodules, the result of hyperplasia of surviving liver cells

● Distortion of normal hepatic lobular architecture and diffuse involvement of the whole liver

🍃 Etiology

● Viral hepatitis
● Chronic alcoholism
● Malnutrition
● Intoxication

第 7 节　肝硬化

🍃 定义

肝硬化是由以下病变导致的肝病

● 肝细胞坏死 长期缓慢进展, 最终导致慢性肝功能衰竭和死亡

● 纤维化 涉及中央静脉和门管区域

● 再生性结节 是存活肝细胞增生的结果

● 整个肝脏弥漫性受累, 最终导致正常肝小叶结构变形

🍃 病因

● 病毒性肝炎
● 慢性酒精中毒
● 营养不良
● 中毒

Pathological Types

- Grossly types
  - Macronodular cirrhosis nodule ＞ 3 mm
  - Micronodular cirrhosis nodule ＜ 3 mm
- Microscopically types
  - Portal cirrhosis
  - Postnecrotic cirrhosis

Clinic-pathologic features

Portal hypertension

Causes

- Sinus obstruction　Extensive liver fibrosis, hepatic sinus occlusion or perisinusoidal fibrosis, blocked portal vein circulation
- Post-sinus obstruction　Pseudolobular compress sublobular veins, blood flow in hepatic sinuses blocked and intervened portal venous blood flow into hepatic sinuses
- Pre-sinus obstruction　small branch of the hepatic artery and portal vein abnormal connect before entering the hepatic sinuses leading arterial high pressure blood into the portal vein

Clinical pathological correlation

Portal hypertension

- Splenomegaly
  - Chronic passive congestion caused

临床分型

- 大体分型
  - 大结节肝硬化＞3毫米
  - 小结节肝硬化＜3毫米

- 镜下分型
  - 门脉性肝硬化
  - 坏死后肝硬化

临床病理特征

门静脉高压症

原因

- **窦性阻塞**　肝内广泛结缔组织增生，肝血窦闭塞或窦周纤维化，门静脉循环受阻

- **窦后性阻塞**　假小叶压迫小叶下静脉，肝血窦内血液流出梗阻，影响门静脉血流入肝血窦

- **窦前性阻塞**　肝动脉小分支和门静脉小分支在汇入肝血窦之前异常吻合，使压力高的动脉血流入门静脉

临床病理联系

门静脉高压

- **脾大**
  - 慢性淤血致脾脏肿大

by the spleen
- Often greater than 500 g
- Ascites
  - Portal hypertension

  - Hypertension of sinus and Disse space
  - Hypoproteinemia decreased osmotic pressure of blood plasma, increased transudation of fluid across the peritoneal membrane
  - Secondary hyperaldosteronism, higher antidiuretic hormone
- Collateral circulation
  - Portal vein→ Stomach coronary vein→ esophageal vein plexus → Azygos vein→precava
  - Portal vein→Mesenteric vein→ rectum vein plexus (hemorrhoid) → iliac vein →postcava
  - Portal vein→umbilical vein→ paraumbilical vein plexus (caput medusae) →abdominal wall vein→precava and postcava
- Gastrointestinal congestion

Hepatic insufficiency
- Protein synthesis disorder Hypoproteinemia
- Clotting factor synthesis disorder Bleeding tendency
- Biliary pigment metabolism

- 常大于500克
- 腹水
  - 门静脉高压致门静脉系统流体静压升高
  - 门静脉高压致肝血窦压升高,血液进入窦周隙
  - 肝功能障碍致合成蛋白质能力下降

  - 灭活醛固酮激素,抗利尿激素水平下降
- 侧支循环形成
  - 门静脉→胃冠状静脉→食管静脉丛→奇静脉→上腔静脉

  - 门静脉→肠系膜静脉→直肠静脉丛(痔疮)→髂静脉→下腔静脉

  - 门静脉→脐静脉→脐旁静脉丛(海蛇头)→腹壁静脉→上、下腔静脉

- 胃肠淤血

肝功能障碍
- 蛋白质合成障碍　低蛋白血症

- 凝血因子合成障碍　出血倾向

- 胆色素代谢障碍　黄疸

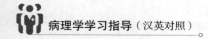

disorder Jaundice

- Hormone inactivation disorder testicular atrophy, male mammary gland development, spider nevus
- Hepatic coma Ammonia and amines from the gastrointestinal tract cannot be detoxified and form pseudoneurotransmitters

Other liver cirrhosis

- Alcoholic liver disease including liver fatty change, alcoholic hepatitis, alcoholic cirrhosis

Section 8　Liver carcinoma

Hepatocellular carcinoma

Etiology

- Aflatoxin B
- Hepatitis B virus infection
- Hepatitis C virus infection
- Liver cirrhosis

Pathological changes

- Grossly　Present as a large solitary mass, or as multiple nodules, or as a diffusely infiltrative lesion
- Microscopically　Tumor is composed of abnormal liver cells of variable differentiation, resembling liver cells arranged in cords separated by

- 对激素灭活作用减弱　睾丸萎缩，男性乳腺发育，蜘蛛痣

- 肝昏迷　来自胃肠道的氨和胺类物质不能被解毒，形成假神经递质

其他肝硬化

- 酒精性肝病包括脂肪肝、酒精性肝炎、酒精性肝硬化

第8节　肝癌

肝细胞癌

病因

- 黄曲霉毒素B
- 乙肝病毒感染
- 丙肝病毒感染
- 肝硬化

病理变化

- 大体　表现为大的孤立肿块，或多发结节，或弥漫性浸润性病变

- 镜下　肿瘤类似肝细胞排列成不规则梁索状，细胞核大，核仁明显，部分细胞质含胆汁

sinusoids. The cells have enlarged nuclei, prominent nucleoli and hyperchromatism and may contain bile in the cytoplasm

Clinical Features

- Hepatocellular carcinoma should be suspected when a patient with known cirrhosis presents with any new symptom such as pain, loss of weight, fever, increasing liver size, or ascites
- Serum AFP is a sensitive marker for hepatocellular carcinoma

Prognosis

- Progression is extremely rapid, and most patients are dead within 1 year
- The median survival after diagnosis is 2 months

Cholangiocarcinoma

- This is a malignant tumor of bile duct origin
- Grossly   Present as a large solitary mass
- Microscopically   Tumor cells arranged as bile duct as irregular glands

临床特征

- 肝硬化患者出现任何新的症状,例如疼痛,体重减轻,发热,肝脏大小增加或腹水时,应怀疑肝细胞癌

- 血清甲胎蛋白(AFP)可作为肝细胞癌检测指标

预后

- 进展非常迅速,大多数患者在1年内死亡
- 诊断后中位生存期为2个月

胆管细胞癌

- 胆管来源的恶性肿瘤

- 大体   常为孤立肿块

- 镜下   肿瘤细胞排列类似胆管,呈不规则腺管状

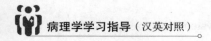

Section 9　Tumors of digestive tract

第9节　消化系统肿瘤

Esophagus carcinoma

Conception

- Esophageal cancer is a malignant tumor from esophagus mucous membrane and gland
- Clinical manifestation is progressive dysphagia

Etiology

- Habit of drinking, eating overheated and coarse food
- There was chronic inflammatory stimulation
- The genetic factors were considered

Pathological feature

- Esophageal cancer often occurs in three physiologic narrow segments, most in the middle narrow part
- Grossly　mucous erosion, rough, ulceration, or mass
- Microscopically　most esophageal carcinoma are squamous cell carcinoma
- Tumor spread　is including tumor cells direct invasion surrounding tissues and metastasis to adjacent lymph nodes

Carcinoma of stomach

Conception

- Gastric cancer is a malignant tumor

食管癌

概述

- 食管癌是由食管黏膜和腺体发生的恶性肿瘤
- 临床表现为进行性吞咽困难

病因

- 长期饮酒，食用过热、过硬及粗糙的食物
- 慢性炎症刺激
- 遗传因素

病理特征

- 食管癌好发于三个生理性狭窄段，以中段最多见
- 大体　可见黏膜糜烂，粗糙，溃疡或肿块
- 镜下　主要为鳞状细胞癌
- 肿瘤扩散　包括直接浸润周围组织及周围淋巴结

胃癌

概述

- 胃癌是由胃黏膜上皮和腺体发生的

from gastric mucous membrane and gland

- It is the second malignant tumor of our country
- Cancer of stomach occurs mostly at gastric lesser curvature of the antrum

Etiology

- Environment and geography Gastric, cancer are frequently found in Asia, such as Japan
- Nitroso compounds in food
- Helicobacter pylori infection
- Chronic inflammatory stimulation for a long time

Histogenesis

- Stem cells in the gastric glands of mucosa neck and bottom of the fovea
- Intestinal metaplasia
- Dysplasia of the gastric mucosa

Pathological features

- Early gastric carcinoma
  ○ Early gastric carcinoma refers to tumor tissue restricted to the mucosa and submucosa of the stomach, with or without lymph node metastasis
  ○ Grossly   As protrude or polypoid, superficial or concave pattern
  ○ Microscopically   most stomach carcinoma are tubular adenocarcinoma and papillary adenocarcinoma

恶性肿瘤

- 占我国恶性肿瘤的第二位

- 好发于胃窦部小弯侧

病因

- 环境地理因素, 亚洲国家如日本多发

- 亚硝基类化合物
- 幽门螺杆菌
- 长期慢性炎症刺激

组织发生

- 胃腺颈部和胃小凹底部干细胞

- 肠上皮化生
- 胃黏膜上皮异型增生

病理特征

- 早期胃癌
  ○ 早期胃癌指肿瘤组织仅限于黏膜及黏膜下层, 无论有无淋巴结转移

  ○ 大体   隆起型或息肉状, 表浅型, 凹陷型
  ○ 镜下   管状腺癌, 乳头状腺癌

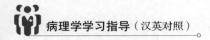

- Advanced gastric carcinoma
  - Grossly There were mucous erosion, ulceration or mass
  - The difference between ulcerative gastric cancer and benign ulcer is that ulcerative gastric cancer showing following features: the shape is irregular and crater-like, the diameter is more than 2 cm, the ulcer is superficial, the edge is uneven, the bottom is convex and concave with necrosis and bleeding, and the surrounding mucosal folds are interrupted and nodular proliferation
  - Sometimes, there is no mass in the presence of diffuse thickening of the gastric wall because of diffuse infiltration, which is called "Linitis plastica"
  - The presence of a large amount of mucous secretion in the tumor tissue looks like semi-transparent jelly called "Colloid carcinoma"
  - Microscopically Gastric cancers mostly are adenocarcinomas including tubular adenocarcinoma, papillary adenocarcinoma, poorly adherent carcinoma (such as signet-ring cell carcinoma) and mixed carcinoma

- 进展期胃癌
  - 大体 可见黏膜糜烂，粗糙，溃疡或肿块
  - 溃疡性胃癌与良性溃疡鉴别在于形状不规则呈火山口样，直径＞2厘米，溃疡表浅，边缘隆起不整齐，底部凹凸不平，有坏死及出血，周围黏膜皱襞中断，呈结节状
  - 有时，肿瘤组织弥漫性浸润可不形成肿块，胃壁弥漫性增厚可不形成肿块，称为"革囊胃"
  - 当癌组织出现大量黏液分泌时呈半透明胶冻状，称为"胶样癌"
  - 镜下 主要为腺癌，包括管状腺癌、乳头状腺癌，低黏附性癌（包括印戒细胞癌）和混合性癌

Spread

- **Direct invade** Tumor cells direct invasion surrounding tissues such as the liver and peritoneum
- **Metastasis**
  ○ Lymphatic metastasis refers to metastasis to the lymph nodes around stomach, and to the left supraclavicular lymph nodes by the thoracic duct in the late stage, which is called Virchow lymph node
  ○ Blood vessels metastasis refers to metastatic nodules in the liver, lung, and other organs
  ○ There was metastatic implantation to the surface of abdominal cavity and pelvic organs. Mucinous or signed-ring cell carcinomas often involve in both ovaries, which is called "Krukenberg tumors"

Prognosis

- The prognosis of gastric cancer almost entirely decided on tumor infiltration depth
- Early gastric cancer are about 85%, the prognosis is good
- The tumor invaded muscle wall but not involving the lymph nodes were about 30%, which have medium prognosis

扩散

- **直接蔓延** 直接浸润周围组织如肝脏和大网膜

- **转移**
  ○ 淋巴道转移指转移至胃周围淋巴结，晚期可经胸导管转移至左锁骨上淋巴结，称为菲尔绍淋巴结

  ○ 血道转移至肝、肺等部位

  ○ 种植性转移至腹腔及盆腔脏器表面。黏液癌或印戒细胞癌常累及双侧卵巢形成克鲁肯贝格瘤

预后

- 预后几乎完全取决于肿瘤的浸润深度

- 早期胃癌占85%，预后较好

- 侵犯肌壁，但未累及淋巴结者占30%，预后中等

- If the stomach wall entirely involved with lymph node metastasis accounted for about 5%, the prognosis is poor

Large Intestine Carcinoma
Conception
- Large intestine carcinoma is a malignant tumor from large intestine mucous membrane and gland, including colonic carcinoma and rectum carcinoma
- It is the third malignant tumor in the world, commonly in western country

Etiology
- Eating diet with high in nutrients and low in fiber
- Chronic hyperplastic lesion of the intestinal mucosa
- Genetic factors familial adenomatous polyposis
- The mechanism of multi-step carcinogenesis of colorectal cancer involves APC-β-catenin pathway, microsatellite instability and CpG island methylation, etc.

Pathological feature
- **Location** Colonic carcinomas are common rectum, sigmoid colon, cecum and ascending colon
- **Grossly** Present as large polypoid masses that project into the lumen,

- 肿瘤胃壁全层并淋巴结转移者约占5%，预后差

大肠癌
概述
- 大肠癌是由大肠黏膜上皮和腺体发生的恶性肿瘤，包括结肠癌和直肠癌

- 全世界第三位恶性肿瘤，西方国家多见

病因
- 饮食习惯为高营养少纤维饮食

- 肠黏膜慢性增生性病变

- 遗传因素有家族性腺瘤性息肉病

- 大肠癌多步癌变机制涉及APC-β-catenin通路，微卫星不稳定性及CpG岛甲基化等

病理特征
- **位置** 直肠最多见，其次为乙状结肠、盲肠升结肠

- **大体** 隆起型、溃疡型、浸润型、胶样型。直肠癌常常为边缘隆起的溃疡

ulceration, infiltrating mass and colloid mass. Rectal carcinomas are most commonly malignant ulcers with raised everted edges

- **Microscopically** Most colon carcinomas are adenocarcinomas including tubular adenocarcinoma, mucous adenocarcinoma, signet-ring cell carcinoma, etc. Squamous cell carcinoma may occur near the rectum and anus

Spread

- **Direct invasion** Surrounding organs, such as the prostate, bladder, and peritoneum
- Metastasis
  - Lymphatic metastases often to regional lymph nodes
  - The blood vessel metastases to the liver, lung and other organs
  - There was implantation metastasis to the surface of internal abdominal organs, and to bilateral ovaries called "Krukenberg tumors "

- **镜下** 主要为腺癌,包括管状腺癌、黏液腺癌、印戒细胞癌等,直肠肛门附近可发生鳞状细胞癌

扩散

- **直接蔓延** 直接浸润周围器官如前列腺、膀胱和腹膜

- **转移**
  - 淋巴道转移常转移至区域淋巴结
  - 血道转移至肝,肺等部位

  - 种植性转移至腹腔内脏器表面,也可转移至双侧卵巢形成克鲁肯贝格瘤

秦 铭 何妙侠

Chapter 9

Diseases of Lymphoid Tissue and Hematopoietic System

第9章

淋巴造血系统疾病

Conception

Organs of the hematopoietic and lymphoid system are mainly including bone marrow, spleen, lymph node, thymus and lymphoid tissue except lymph node

概述

淋巴造血系统包括骨髓、脾、淋巴结、胸腺及结外淋巴组织

Section 1　Benign lesion of lymph node

第1节　淋巴结良性病变

Structure of lymph node

- Lymph node is discrete encapsulated nodule, usually ovoid and ranging in diameter from a few millimeters to several centimeters
- Parenchyma of lymph node is composed of the cortex and the medulla
- The cortex is composed of superficial cortex containing nodules of B-lymphocytes; the paracortex of T-cell-dependent region; and cortical

淋巴结结构

- 淋巴结为大小不一的圆形或椭圆形灰红色结节

- 淋巴结分为皮质和髓质两部分

- 皮质由含淋巴小结的皮质区(B细胞区)、副皮质区(T细胞区)和皮质淋巴窦构成,髓质由髓索和髓窦组成

sinuses. The medulla contains medullary cords and medullary sinuses

- The follicles of the lymph node cortex consist of germinal center, mantle cell and marginal area. The cells in the germinal center are mixed and arranged in polar direction, and starry sky can be seen in the germinal center

- 淋巴结皮质淋巴滤泡由生发中心、套区和边缘区构成,生发中心由混合细胞构成,排列有极向,可见星空现象

Reactive hyperplasia of lymph node

Pathologic changes

- Grossly
  - Lymph nodes are soft, slightly enlarged
  - Usually 1～2 cm in diameter, with smooth capsule
  - A gray-red or gray-white of cut surface
- Microscopically
  - The lymph node structure is preserved
  - hyperplasia of lymphoid follicle　Big and more follicle
  - Paracortical lymphoid hyperplasia　Paracortex area become lager and widen
  - Sinus histiocytosis　Distention and prominence of the lymphatic sinus and the lining macrophages Hyperplasia
  - Three patterns mix together

淋巴结反应性增生

病理变化

- **大体**
  - 淋巴结软,稍肿大
  - 通常直径1～2厘米,包膜完整
  - 切面灰红色或灰白色
- **镜下**
  - 淋巴结结构存在
  - **淋巴滤泡增生**　滤泡大且增多
  - **副皮质区增生**　副皮质区淋巴细胞增生,皮质旁区域增宽
  - **窦组织胞增生**　淋巴窦扩张,其内组织细胞增生
  - 三种形式混合增生

Infectious disease of lymph node

- The common infectious diseases of lymph node are tuberculosis, cat scratch disease and infectious mononucleosis, which are caused by tuberculosis, Bartonella Hansel and Epstein-Barr virus infection, respectively
- Cat scratch disease
  ○ Cat scratch disease is an infectious disease
  ○ Bartonella henselae is the etiologic agent, always appeared after one to two weeks by cat scratch
  ○ It commonly involved axillary and cervical lymph nodes
  ○ Microscopically The epithelioid cells form a granuloma, and the neutrophils form a micro-abscess in the center
  ○ It is the limitations of the benign self-limiting disease

Section 2   Lymphoid neoplasm: lymphoma

Conception

Location

- Lymphoma   lymph node, extra lymph node

淋巴结感染性疾病

- 淋巴结常见感染性疾病包括结核,猫抓病和传染性单核细胞增多症,分别由结核杆菌、汉赛巴尔通体和EB病毒感染引起
- 猫抓病
  ○ 猫抓病是一种感染性疾病
  ○ 病原体为汉赛巴尔通体,常在猫抓后1～2周出现
  ○ 常常累及腋下和颈部淋巴结
  ○ 镜下　为上皮样细胞形成肉芽肿,中央可见中性粒细胞形成微脓肿
  ○ 为良性自限性局限性疾病

第2节　淋巴组织肿瘤：淋巴瘤

概述

位置

- 淋巴瘤　发生于淋巴结、结外淋巴组织

- Leukemia Bone marrow and peripheral blood
- Myeloma Bone marrow

Classifications

- Hodgkin's lymphoma (HL)
- Non-Hodgkin's lymphoma (NHL)
  - Precursor cell lymphoma
  - Mature cell lymphoma

Immunophenotype

- Myeloid cell neoplasm
  - Acute myeloid leukemia myeloid cell clonal proliferation in bone marrow
  - Chronic myeloid leukemia the Philadelphia chromosome t(9; 22) (q34; q11), BCR-ABL gene fusion and translocation
- Lymphoid cell neoplasm
  - B cell lymphoma B cell markers are CD19, CD20, CD79a and PAX5
  - T cell lymphoma T cell markers are CD2, CD3, CD4, CD5, CD7 and CD8
  - T/NK cell lymphoma Express T cell and NK cell markers, the NK cell marker is CD56
- Histiocytic neoplasm
  - Follicular dendritic cell sarcoma expresses CD21, CD23, and CD35
  - Langerhans cell histiocytosis

- 白血病 累及骨髓和外周血

- 骨髓瘤 累及骨髓

分类

- 霍奇金淋巴瘤（HL）
- 非霍奇金淋巴瘤（NHL）
  - 前体细胞淋巴瘤
  - 成熟细胞淋巴瘤

免疫表型

- 髓系肿瘤
  - 急性髓系白血病 骨髓原始细胞克隆性增生
  - 慢性髓系白血病 出现费城染色体t（9；22）（q34；q11），BCR-ABL基因融合

- 淋巴瘤
  - B细胞淋巴瘤 B细胞标记包括CD19，CD20，CD79a和PAX5
  - T细胞淋巴瘤 T细胞标记包括CD2，CD3，CD4，CD5，CD7和CD8等
  - T/NK细胞淋巴瘤 表达T细胞及NK细胞标记，NK细胞标记是CD56
- 组织细胞肿瘤
  - 滤泡树突细胞肉瘤 表达CD21，CD23，CD35
  - 朗格汉斯细胞组织细胞增生

expresses CD1a, S100, and Langerin

- ○ Mast cell tumor   expresses CD117

Hodgkin's lymphoma (HL)

Basic features

- Accounts for 10% ～ 20% of all lymphomas
- The tumor located lymph nodes
- The tumor spreads gradually from one or a group of lymph nodes
- There are only a few neoplastic large cells (Classical R–S cells) in tumor tissue, accounting for only 0.1% ～ 10% of all cells
- There are often reactive cells with varying numbers, mainly small lymphocytes and eosinophils in the background
- According to morphological characteristics, HL can be divided into nodular lymphocytic dominant HL and classic HL
- It is believed that tumor cells of HL are derived from B lymphocytes
- The prognosis is better than NHL

Pathological changes

- Grossly
    - ○ lymph nodes are enlarged, with a smooth surface
    - ○ The cut surface is usually homogeneously with yellow-white

症　表达CD1a, S-100, Langerin

- ○ 肥大细胞肿瘤　表达CD117

霍奇金淋巴瘤（HL）

基本特征

- 占所有淋巴瘤的10%～20%
- 肿瘤发生于淋巴结
- 肿瘤从一个或一组淋巴结开始逐渐扩散
- 肿瘤组织中只有少数肿瘤性大细胞（特征性里-施细胞），仅占所有细胞的0.1%～10%
- 病变背景常有数量不等的反应性细胞，主要为小淋巴细胞、嗜酸性粒细胞等
- 根据形态学特征分为结节性淋巴细胞为主型HL和经典型HL
- 大部分观点认为肿瘤细胞来源于B淋巴细胞
- 预后相对于NHL较好

病理变化

- 大体
    - ○ 淋巴结肿大，表面光滑
    - ○ 切面均质，常见黄白色坏死

necrotic focus

- Microscopically
  - Structure of lymph node damaged partially or completely, which is replaced by tumor tissue
  - Neoplastic cell: large with two or more nucleus, the specific feature is that these tumor cell always have prominent eosinophilic large nucleoli, which is called as R-S cell
  - R-S cell variant including popcorn-like cell (multilobate nuclei), lacunar cell (abundant pale cytoplasm) and Hodgkin cell (mononucleate tumor giant cell)
  - There are numerous lymphocytes, eosinophilia neutrophil, plasma cells and histiocytes among tumor cells in the background

Classification

- Nodular lymphocyte predominant Hodgkin's lymphoma (NLPHL), the tumor cell is CD30–, CD15– and CD20+
- Classic Hodgkin's lymphoma (CHL), including nodular sclerosis CHL. mixed cellularity CHL, lymphocytic rich CHL, lymphocytic depletion CHL, the tumor cell is CD30+, CD15+/– and CD20–
- The most common type is nodular

- 镜下
  - 淋巴结结构部分或完全破坏,被肿瘤组织取代

  - 肿瘤细胞:较大,有两个或两个以上细胞核,肿瘤细胞有突出的嗜酸性大核仁,称为里-施细胞

  - 里-施细胞变型包括爆米花样细胞(多叶状细胞核)、腔隙细胞(含丰富细胞质)和霍奇金细胞(单核肿瘤巨细胞)

  - 肿瘤组织背景中有大量淋巴细胞、嗜酸性粒细胞、浆细胞和组织细胞等

分类

- 结节性淋巴细胞为主型霍奇金淋巴瘤,肿瘤细胞呈$CD30^-$,$CD15^-$,$CD20^+$

- 经典型霍奇金淋巴瘤,包括结节硬化型,混合细胞型,淋巴细胞丰富型,淋巴细胞减少型,肿瘤细胞呈$CD30^+$,$CD15^{+/-}$,$CD20^-$

- 最常见的类型是结节硬化型经典型

sclerosis classic Hodgkin's lymphoma

Clinical features and prognosis

- Clinical features
  - HL always involving children and young adults
  - Tumors often start in a lymph node, gradually spread to another site, such as begin with cervical lymph nodes, followed by mediastinal, axillary and inguinal lymph nodes
  - Presents with painless, progressive lymphadenopathy
  - There are 4 stages according to the range of lymph node involvement, staging of HL was made according to Ann Arbor staging
- Prognosis
  - Most patients of HL have a good prognosis
  - The chemotherapy regimen for HL is usually by ABVD, and the patient response to the treatment is good

🌿 Non-Hodgkin's lymphoma (NHL)

Basic features

- NHL accounts for 80%～90% of all lymphomas
- Location: Two-thirds occur in lymph nodes, 1/3 occurs outside lymph nodes, such as gastrointestinal tract and skin

霍奇金淋巴瘤

临床特征及预后

- 临床特征
  - 霍奇金淋巴瘤主要发生于儿童及年轻人
  - 肿瘤常从一个淋巴结开始，逐渐扩散到另一个部位，如从颈部淋巴结开始，其次是纵隔、腋窝和腹股沟淋巴结
  - 表现为无痛、进行性淋巴结肿大
  - 按安娜堡分期进行HL临床分期，可根据淋巴结受累范围分为4个分期
- 预后
  - 大部分霍奇金淋巴瘤病人预后较好
  - 常用化疗方案为ABVD，病人治疗反应均较好

🌿 非霍奇金淋巴瘤（NHL）

基本特征

- NHL占所有淋巴瘤的80%～90%
- 位置：2/3发生于淋巴结，1/3发生于淋巴结外，如胃肠道、皮肤等部位

- According to the different cell origin, they are divided into B, T, T/NK cell tumors
- The NHL is classified into progenitor cells and mature cells tumor according to their developmental extent
- Tumors are classified as indolent or invasive according to their biological behavior
- The most common tumor of NHL in lymph nodes is diffuse large B-cell lymphoma
- The most common extranodal tumor is mucosa-associated extranodal marginal zone lymphoma
- NHL tumor tissue is mainly composed of tumor cells and fewer background cells
- Tumor cells were more uniform in B-cell lymphoma than in T-cell lymphoma

Pathologic changes

- Grossly
  - Involved lymph nodes enlargement
  - The cut surface is homogeneous, yellow-white to gray
  - The consistency varies from soft to moderately firm. Necrotic focus can be seen
- Microscopically
  - Structure of lymph node is

- 根据细胞起源不同分为B、T、T/NK细胞肿瘤

- 根据细胞发育程度分为前体细胞性和成熟细胞性

- 根据肿瘤生物学行为分为惰性和侵袭性

- 淋巴结最常见的肿瘤是弥漫性大B细胞淋巴瘤

- 淋巴结外最常见的肿瘤是黏膜相关组织结外边缘区淋巴瘤

- NHL肿瘤组织中肿瘤细胞占主要成分,间质细胞较少

- 相对于T细胞淋巴瘤,B细胞淋巴瘤中肿瘤细胞较一致

病理变化

- 大体
  - 受累淋巴结肿大
  - 切面均匀,黄白色至灰色
  - 质地从软到中等不等,可见坏死灶
- 镜下
  - 淋巴结结构完全消失,被肿瘤组

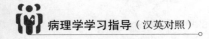
disappeared completely, which is replaced by tumor tissue

- A predominant population of tumor cells effaced the lymph node architecture, the tumor cell is consistent
- Tumor cells arranged diffusely or arranged as nodular structure
- Tumor cells infiltrate into capsule of lymph node and extra-nodular tissue

Common types of Non-Hodgkin's lymphoma

Follicular lymphoma

- Follicular lymphoma always involving adult
- Origin from germinal center B cell
- Nodular growth pattern
- Tumor follicle composed of centrocyte and centroblast, it is classified to 3 grades by the numbers of centroblast in HPF
- B-cell marker positive CD19, CD20, CD10 (+)
- Bcl-2 (+) can help to distinguish between reactive and neoplastic follicle
- Most tumor has t (14;18) IGH/BCL2 translocation

织取代

- 肿瘤细胞较一致，均匀一致破坏淋巴结结构

- 肿瘤细胞呈弥漫性或结节状排列

- 肿瘤细胞浸润淋巴结包膜以及结外淋巴组织

常见非霍奇金淋巴瘤

滤泡性淋巴瘤

- 多累及成人

- 生发中心B细胞来源
- 结节状生长模式
- 肿瘤滤泡由中心细胞和中心母细胞构成，根据中心母细胞数量分为1～3级

- B细胞标记CD19、CD20、CD10阳性（+）

- Bcl-2（+）有助于区分反应性滤泡和肿瘤性滤泡

- 大部分有t（14；18）IGH/BCL2易位

Diffuse large B-cell lymphoma (DLBCL)

- DLBCL constitutes 25% ～ 35% of adult non-Hodgkin lymphomas in developed countries, and a higher percentage in developing countries
- It is more common in elderly individuals
- DLBCL is a neoplasm of medium or large B lymphoid cells whose nuclei are the same size as, or larger than those of normal macrophages, or more than twice the size of those of normal lymphocytes, with a diffuse growth pattern
- DLBCL can be subdivided into germinal centre B-cell (GCB) subtype and activated B-cell (ABC) subtype
- Patients may present with nodal or extranodal disease, usually with a rapidly enlarging tumour mass at single or multiple nodal or extranodal sites
- Lymph nodes demonstrate partial or more commonly total architectural effacement by a diffuse proliferation of medium or large lymphoid cells
- B-cell marker positive CD19 and CD20
- It is an aggressive lymphoma, but sensitive to chemotherapy, the regime

弥漫性大B细胞淋巴瘤（DLBCL）

- DLBCL占发达国家成人非霍奇金淋巴瘤的25%～35%，在发展中国家比例更高
- 多见于老年人
- DLBCL是一种中至大的B细胞淋巴瘤，其细胞核大小与正常巨噬细胞相同或大于正常巨噬细胞，或核大小为正常淋巴细胞的两倍以上，呈弥漫性生长
- DLBCL可分为生发中心B细胞（GCB）亚型和活化B细胞（ABC）亚型
- 患者可表现为淋巴结或淋巴结外病变，通常为单个或多个淋巴结或结外其他部位肿瘤迅速增大
- 淋巴结结构大部分消失，代之以弥漫性增生的肿瘤细胞
- B细胞标记阳性如CD19、CD20
- DLBCL侵袭性淋巴瘤，但对化疗较敏感，采用CHOP方案和抗CD20单

is CHOP and anti-CD20 shows better response in treatment

Burkitt lymphoma (BL)

- Burkitt lymphoma is a highly aggressive but curable lymphoma that often presents in extranodal sites
- BL is the most common childhood malignancy
- The jaws and other facial bone, distal ileum and caecum are frequently involved. It is associated with EBV infection
- There are three types: Endemic BL, Sporadic BL and Immunodeficiency-associated BL
- The tumour cells are medium sized and show a diffuse monotonous pattern of growth. The cells appear to be cohesive but often exhibit squared-off borders of retracted cytoplasm
- A so-called starry sky pattern is usually present, which is due to the presence of numerous tingible body macrophages. The tumour has an extremely high proliferation rate
- The molecular hallmark of BL is the translocation of *MYC* at band 8q24 to the *IGH* region on chromosome 14q32, t (8;14)(q24;q32)
- BL is a highly aggressive but potentially curable tumour; intensive

抗治疗效果较好

伯基特淋巴瘤（BL）

- 伯基特淋巴瘤是一种侵袭性强但可治愈的淋巴瘤,常发生于结外部位
- 伯基特淋巴瘤是儿童最常见的恶性肿瘤
- 常累及颌骨等面骨、回肠远端及盲肠,与EBV感染有关
- 有三种类型:地方性BL、偶发BL和免疫缺陷相关BL
- BL由单形性中等大小B细胞组成,胞质嗜碱性,核分裂象多,异型性明显,呈镶嵌状排列
- 可见星空现象,与存在较多具有吞噬现象的巨噬细胞有关,肿瘤细胞增殖指数高
- BL分子标志是*MYC*和*IGH*基因易位t（8；14）（q24；q32）
- BL是高度侵袭性但可治愈的肿瘤,70%～90%病例强化化疗可长期存

chemotherapy leads to long-term overall survival in 70% ~ 90% of cases, with children doing better than adults

活，儿童预后比成人好

Extranodal NK/T cell lymphoma

结外NK/T细胞淋巴瘤

- Extranodal NK/T cell lymphoma is a predominantly extranodal lymphoma of NK-cell or T-cell lineage

- 结外NK/T细胞淋巴瘤，鼻型主要为NK细胞或T细胞来源的结外淋巴瘤

- It is more prevalent in Asians and association with EB virus

- 亚洲人多见，与EBV感染有关

- The upper aerodigestive tract (nasal cavity, nasopharynx, paranasal sinuses, and palate) is most commonly involved

- 最常见于上呼吸道（鼻腔、鼻咽、副鼻窦和上颚）

- It is characterized by vascular damage and destruction, prominent necrosis. The cytological spectrum is very broad with cytotoxic phenotype

- 形态特点是血管损伤和破坏，明显坏死，肿瘤细胞形态多样，表达细胞毒性表型

- The most typical immunophenotype of tumor cells is $CD3^+$, $CD2^+$, $CD5^-$, $CD56^+$, and positive to cytotoxic molecules

- 肿瘤细胞最典型的免疫表型为$CD3^+$、$CD2^+$、$CD5^-$、$CD56^+$，对细胞毒性分子呈阳性

- It is highly aggressive, with short survival and poor response to therapy

- 肿瘤高侵袭性，生存期短，对治疗反应差

何妙侠

Chapter 10

Diseases of Urinary System

Conception

Functions of kidney

- Excretes the waste products of metabolism
- Precisely regulates the body's concentration of water and salt
- Maintains the appropriate acid-alkaline balance of plasma
- Serves as an endocrine organ: erythropoietin, renin, prostaglandin

Renal structure

- The kidney is composed of nephrons and collecting ducts, the nephrons are composed of glomerulus and tubules
- Filtering membrane
  - Endothelial cells (EC) A thin layer of fenestrated EC fenestrum, 70 ～ 100 nm in diameter, with negative electric charge and sialoglycoprotein on the surface
  - Glomerular basement membrane

第10章

泌尿系统疾病

概述

肾脏的功能

- 排出新陈代谢的废物

- 精确调节人体中水和盐的浓度

- 维持血浆中适当的酸碱平衡

- 具有内分泌功能：促红细胞生成素，肾素，前列腺素

肾脏的结构

- 肾脏由肾单位和集合管组成，其中肾单位由肾小球和肾小管组成

- 滤过膜
  - 内皮细胞 薄层有窗孔的内皮细胞，窗孔直径70～100纳米，表面为唾液酸糖蛋白，带负电荷

  - 肾小球基底膜 由内疏松层、致

(GBM) GBM is composed of Lamina sparse interna (thin), Lamina densa (thick) and Lamina sparse externa (thin)

密层和外疏松层构成

- Podocyte Visceral epithelial cell
- Filtering membrane Highly specialized podocytes form the outer layer of the filtration membrane, adjacent foot processes form filtration slit with negative electric charge and sialoglycoprotein on the surface

- 足细胞 肾小球脏层上皮细胞
- 滤过膜构成 高度特化的足细胞构成滤过膜的外层，相邻足突之间为滤过隙，足细胞表面为唾液酸糖蛋白，带负电荷

- Mesangium
  - Mesangial cell Contraction, phagocytosis, producing matrix and collagen, secreting a number of cytokines
  - Mesangial matrix
- Renal capsule
- Glomerular barrier function
  - Water and small solutes can pass through the glomerular filtration membrane
  - Large molecular proteins are almost impossible
  - Whether they can pass depends on their size and charge

- 系膜
  - 系膜细胞 收缩，吞噬，合成基质和胶原蛋白，分泌多种细胞因子

  - 系膜基质
- 肾球囊
- 肾小球屏障功能
  - 水和小分子溶质可以通过肾小球滤过膜

  - 大分子蛋白质几乎不能通过肾小球滤过膜
  - 能否通过取决于他们的体积和携带电荷

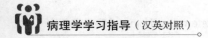
Section 1　Glomerular diseases

Conception

Glomerulonephritis (GN)

- It is a group of diseases mainly caused by glomerular injury and lesion, there are two types of GN

- Primary glomerulonephritis: Immune mechanisms

- Secondary glomerulonephritis: SLE, hypertension, diabetes and so on

Etiology and pathogenesis

The main cause of GN is antigen-antibody reaction

- Antigen origin
  - Endogenous Ag
    - Glomerular Ag, including GBM Ag, Foot process Ag, Membrane of EC
    - Non-glomerular Ag, including DNA, Immunoglobulin, Tumor Ag
  - Exogenous Ag
    Including bacterium, virus, parasite, fungus, drugs, foreign serum
- Ag-Ab complexes
  - Immune complex deposition *in situ*
    - The antibody reacts directly

第1节　肾小球疾病

概述

肾小球肾炎（GN）

- 是以肾小球损伤和病变为主的一组疾病,有两型

- 原发性肾小球肾炎：免疫机制

- 继发性肾小球肾炎：系统性红斑狼疮,高血压,糖尿病等

病因与发病机制

GN主要原因是抗原抗体反应

- 抗原来源
  - 内源性抗原
    - 肾小球性抗原,包括肾小球基底膜抗原,足突抗原,内皮细胞膜抗原
    - 非肾小球性抗原,包括脱氧核糖核酸,免疫球蛋白,肿瘤抗原
  - 外源性抗原
    包括细菌,病毒,寄生虫,真菌,药物,外源性血清
- 抗原抗体复合物
  - 原位免疫复合物沉积
    - 抗体直接与肾小球的抗原成分

with the antigen component of the glomerulus or the antigen implanted into the glomerulus through blood circulation, forming an *in situ* immune complex in the glomerulus, causing glomerular lesions

或经血液循环植入肾小球的抗原反应,在肾小球内形成原位免疫复合物,引起肾小球病变

- ○ Anti-GBM nephritis (Masugi's nephritis)
  - This type of nephritis is caused by the reaction of antibodies with the antigenic component of the glomerular basement membrane itself

○ 抗肾小球基膜抗体引起的肾炎
  - 由抗体与肾小球基膜本身的抗原成分反应引起

- Circulating immune complex deposition
  ○ Exogenous Ag combined Ab deposited the glomerulus from blood
  ○ Deposit locations are including mesangial region, subendothelial, subepithelial area
  ○ There are granular deposits at the site of glomerular lesions
  ○ There accompany with immunoglobins, complements and microphages
  ○ The important factors are the size of immune complex molecules and the charge they carry on

- 循环免疫复合物沉积
  ○ 外源性抗原与抗体结合通过血液沉积于肾小球
  ○ 沉积的部位包括系膜区、上皮下和内皮下
  ○ 肾小球病变部位有颗粒状沉积物
  ○ 常伴随补体激活、免疫球蛋白和巨噬细胞
  ○ 最重要的因素是免疫复合物分子的大小和免疫复合物携带的电荷

- Immune complex deposition in situ
  Antibodies react directly with the antigenic components of the glomeruli

- 原位免疫复合物沉积
  是抗体直接与肾小球本身的抗原成分或经血液循环植入肾小球的抗原

themselves or the antigens that are inserted into the glomeruli through the blood circulation to form an in situ immune complex in the glomeruli

○ Anti-glomerular basement membrane antibodies related Nephritis

- Formation of GBM Ag
- Structural changes of membrane
- Cross-reaction because of the same Ag with organism
- Fluorescence Ab deposition in the GBM as continuous linear pattern

○ Heymann nephritis

- Heymann nephritis is a classic model for the study of primary membranous glomerulopathy in humans
- This model uses the proximal convoluted tubule brush border component as an antigen to generate antibodies in mice and cause lesions similar to human membranous glomerulopathy
- Numerous electron-dense deposits between epithelium and basement membrane (subepithelial) Granular deposits

○ Ab against planted Ag

- Ab react in situ with previously "planted" non-glomerular Ag

发生反应,在肾小球内形成原位免疫复合物

○ 抗肾小球基底膜抗体引起的肾炎

- 肾小球基底膜抗原的形成
- 肾小球基底膜结构的变化
- 抗原与微生物的交叉反应

- GBM可见荧光抗体呈连续的线性沉积

○ 海曼肾炎

- 海曼肾炎是人类研究原发性膜性肾小球病的经典模型

- 该模型以近曲小管刷状缘成分为抗原,使小鼠产生抗体,引起与人膜性肾小球肾病相似的病变

- 上皮和基底膜之间的大量电子致密沉积物(上皮下)

○ 抗体与植入抗原反应

- Ab与先前"植入"的非肾小球Ag原位反应

- The planted Ag is cationic molecules or proteins or DNA、bacterial products、large aggregated protein (such as aggregated IgG)、virus, parasitic product and drugs
- Granular or heterogeneous pattern of Ig deposits

○ Pathogenesis of glomerulus injury

Activation of alternative complement pathway

- The products of complement activated such as C3a,C5a and infiltration of neutrophil and monocyte

Anti-glomerular cell Ab without IC deposits

- Ab directed to glomerular cell Ag→ direct cell injury
- Ab to mesangial cell Ag→ mesangiolysis, mesangial proliferation
- Ab to Endothelial cells Ag → thrombosis

Cell mediated immunity

- Sensitized T cells cause glomerular injury
- Inflammatory mediator such as macrophage, monocyte, platelets and other cytokines and chemokines

- 植入的抗原为阳离子分子或蛋白质、脱氧核糖核酸、细菌产物、大的聚集蛋白（例如聚集IgG）、病毒、寄生虫产物、药物等

- 沉积物为颗粒或非均质性免疫球蛋白沉积物

○ 肾小球损伤的病理机制

补体活化途径

- 补体活化产物如C3a, C5a, 常伴随炎细胞如中性粒细胞、单核细胞浸润

抗肾小球细胞抗体作用

- 针对肾小球细胞Ag的抗体→直接损伤细胞
- 针对肾小球系膜细胞Ag的抗体→肾小球系膜溶解，系膜增生
- 针对内皮细胞Ag的抗体→血栓形成

细胞介导的免疫

- 致敏T细胞引起肾小球损伤

- 炎症介质包括巨噬细胞、单核细胞、血小板等其他细胞因子、化学因子等

Basic pathological changes

- Glomerular hypercellularity
  - Cell Proliferation
    Mesangial cells, Endothelial cells, Parietal epithelial cells
  - Inflammatory cell infiltration
    Neutrophils, Lymphocytes, Monocytes
- GBM thickening mesangial matrix increasing
- Inflammatory exudation and necrosis
  - Exudation   neutrophil, fibrin
  - Necrosis   fibrinous necrosis
- Hyalinization and sclerosis
- Renal tubules and interstitial changes
  - The renal tubules epithelial cells degeneration
  - Protein cast
  - Interstitial inflammation cell infiltration
- Nomenclature of glomerular injury
  - Diffuse   involving all or majority of glomeruli (＞50%)
  - Focal   involving a certain proportion of glomeruli (＜50%)
  - Global   involving the entire glomerulus or large part of each glomerulus (＞50%)
  - Segmental   affecting a part of each glomerulus (＜50%)

Clinical manifestation

- Acute nephritic syndrome
  - Hematuria, proteinuria, oliguria

基本病理变化

- 肾小球细胞增多
  - 细胞增生
    系膜细胞,内皮细胞,壁上皮细胞
  - 炎细胞浸润
    中性粒细胞,淋巴细胞,单核细胞
- 基底膜增厚,肾小球系膜基质增多

- 炎性渗出和坏死
  - 渗出   中性粒细胞,纤维蛋白
  - 坏死   纤维性坏死
- 玻璃样变和硬化
- 肾小管和肾间质改变
  - 肾小管上皮细胞变性

  - 蛋白管型
  - 间质炎细胞浸润
- 肾小球损伤的命名
  - 弥漫性   累及全部或大部分肾小球(＞50%)
  - 局灶性   涉及一定比例的肾小球(＜50%)
  - 球性   涉及整个肾小球或每个肾小球的大部分(＞50%)

  - 节段性   影响每个肾小球的一部分(＜50%)

临床表现

- 急性肾炎综合征
  - 血尿,蛋白尿,少尿

- ○ Edema
- ○ Hypertension
- ○ Severe azotemia
- Rapidly progressive nephritic syndrome
  - ○ Hematuria, Proteinuria, Oliguria or Anuria
  - ○ Edema
  - ○ Azotemia, acute renal failure
- Nephrotic syndrome
  - ○ Heavy proteinuria ($\geqslant 3.5$ g)
  - ○ Severe edema
  - ○ Hypoalbuminemia (< 30 g/L)
  - ○ Hyperlipidemia and lipiduria
- Asymptomatic hematuria or proteinuria
  - ○ Continuous or recurrent hematuria (macroscopic or microscopic)
  - ○ Mild proteinuria
- Chronic nephritic syndrome
  - ○ Polyuria nocturia
  - ○ low specific gravity urine
  - ○ Hypertension
  - ○ Azotemia and uremia
  - ○ Anemia

Pathological types
- Acute diffuse proliferative GN
- Rapidly progressive GN (RPGN)
- Membranous GN
- Minimal change GN
- Focal segmental GN

- ○ 水肿
- ○ 高血压
- ○ 严重时氮质血症
- 快速进行性肾病综合征
  - ○ 血尿,蛋白尿,少尿或无尿
  - ○ 水肿
  - ○ 氮质血症,急性肾功能衰竭
- 肾病综合征(三高一低)
  - ○ 高蛋白尿($\geqslant 3.5$克)
  - ○ 严重水肿
  - ○ 低白蛋白血症(< 30克/升)
  - ○ 高脂血症和脂尿
- 无症状性血尿或蛋白尿
  - ○ 连续或复发性血尿(肉眼或镜下)
  - ○ 轻度蛋白尿
- 慢性肾炎综合征
  - ○ 夜尿症
  - ○ 低比重尿
  - ○ 高血压
  - ○ 氮质血症和尿毒症
  - ○ 贫血

病理类型
- 急性弥漫性增生性肾小球肾炎
- 急进性肾小球肾炎(RPGN)
- 膜性肾小球肾炎
- 微小病变性肾小球肾炎
- 局灶性节段性肾小球肾炎

- Membranoproliferative GN
- Mesangial proliferative GN
- IgA nephropathy
- Chronic glomerulonephritis

Type 1　Acute diffuse proliferative glomerulonephritis (GN)

Conception

- Also known as Endocapillary proliferative GN
- Since most cases are related to infection, it is also called postinfectious GN, which can be divided into poststreptococcal GN and nonstreptococcal GN
- It is characterized by proliferation of endothelial cells and mesangial cells, with infiltration of neutrophils and macrophages

Etiology and pathogenesis

- Main factors
  - Most common: Group A β-hemolytic streptococci type 12. 4. 1
  - Others: pneumococci, staphylococcus hepatitis B virus (HBV)
- Immune mediated disease
  - Immune complex depositing
  - Anti-o Ab↑
  - Serum complement level↓
- Pathological changes
  - Grossly
    - Enlarge

- 膜增生性肾小球肾炎
- 系膜增生性肾小球肾炎
- IgA肾病
- 慢性肾小球肾炎

类型1　急性弥漫性增生性肾小球肾炎

概述

- 又叫毛细血管内增生性肾小球肾炎
- 由于大多数病例与感染有关,也称感染后性肾小球肾炎,分为链球菌感染后性肾小球肾炎和非链球菌感染性肾小球肾炎
- 特点是内皮细胞和系膜细胞增生,伴中性粒细胞和巨噬细胞浸润

病因与发病机制

- 主要因素
  - 最常见的是A族乙型溶血性链球菌中的12、4、1型
  - 其他:肺炎球菌,葡萄球菌,乙型肝炎病毒（HBV）
- 免疫介导性因素
  - 免疫复合物沉积增加
  - 抗"O"抗体增加
  - 血清补体水平下降
- 病理改变
  - 大体
    - 增大

- Dark red
- Petechial hemorrhage
- flea-biting kidney
○ Microscopically
- **Glomeruli** Enlarged glomeruli, hypercellularity
- **Proliferative cells** Endothelial, Mesangial cells
- **Infiltrative cell** Neutrophil, Macrophage
- **Bloodless of glomeruli** Proliferating of EC and Mesangial cell; Swelling of EC; Obliterate capillary lumens; Blood supply and GFR decreased; Capillary wall segmental fibrinous necrosis causes hematuria
- **Renal tubules** Proximal tubule epithelial cell degeneration; Tubules contains protein or RBC casts
- **Renal interstitium** Congestion; Edema; Inflammatory cell infiltration
○ Immunofluorescence
- There are granular fluorescence deposits in GBM and mesangium, including IgG, IgM and C3
○ Electronic Microscopically
- "Humps" electron-dense deposits
- commonly between subepithelial

- 暗红
- 粟粒大小的出血点
- 跳蚤肾
○ 光镜
- **肾小球** 肾小球增大, 细胞过多
- **增生的细胞** 内皮细胞, 系膜细胞
- **浸润的细胞** 中性粒细胞; 巨噬细胞
- **肾小球缺血** 内皮细和系膜细胞的增生; 内皮细胞肿胀; 毛细血管腔闭塞; 血流量减少导致肾小球滤过率减小; 节段性纤维素样坏死导致血尿
- **肾小管** 近端小管上皮细胞变性; 小管含有蛋白质或红细胞形成管型
- **肾间质** 淤血; 浮肿; 炎性细胞浸润
○ 免疫荧光
- 免疫荧光显示GBM和系膜颗粒荧光沉积, 包括IgG、IgM和C3
○ 电镜
- "驼峰"样电子致密沉积物
- 通常上皮细胞下和基底膜之间

cells and GBM

- subendothelial cells
- intramembrane

Clinical-Pathological Features

Acute nephritic syndrome

- The changes of urine
  - Hematuria, proteinuria bloodless glomeruli, making GFR declining
  - Oliguria Proliferation of cells and swelling of EC
- Edema
  - Glomerular filtration rate decreased and causes depositing of water and sodium
  - Hypersensitivity reaction causes capillary permeability increased
- Hypertension Increased blood volume due to sodium and water retention

Prognosis

- Children good prognosis
  - More than 95% can recovered
  - Less than 1% develop a rapidly progressive glomerulonephritis
  - 1%～2% change to chronic GN
- In adults poorly prognosis
  - 60% patient could recover
  - Some patients develop rapidly progressive GN
  - Some patients develop chronic GN

- 内皮下细胞
- 基底膜内

临床病理特征

急性肾炎综合征

- 尿液的变化
  - 血尿、蛋白尿　毛细血管壁的损伤会增加滤过膜的通透性，从而导致血尿和蛋白尿
  - 少尿　细胞增殖和基底膜肿胀导致肾小球缺血，使肾小球滤过率下降
- 水肿
  - 肾小球滤过率下降导致水钠潴留
  - 超敏反应导致毛细血管通透性升高
- 高血压　水钠潴留导致血容量增加

结局

- 儿童　预后良好
  - ＞95%患者可以完全恢复
  - ＜1%发展为快速进行性肾小球肾炎
  - 1%～2%转成慢性肾小球肾炎
- 成人　预后不良
  - 60%可以恢复
  - 部分发展为急进性肾小球肾炎
  - 部分发展为慢性肾小球肾炎

Type 2　Acute Rapidly progressive glomerulonephritis (RPGN)

Conception

- Characterized by Parietal epithelial cells of glomerular proliferation form crescent
- Also called crescentic GN

Pathogenesis and classification

- Most cases are caused by immune mechanisms, which can be divided into three types according to pathology and immunology
- RPGN　anti-GBM nephritis
  ○ Immunofluorescence
    - linear deposits of IgG and C3
    - Anti-GBM antibody cross-reacts with alveolar basement membrane
  ○ Clinical manifestation　Goodpasture syndrome
    - Pulmonary hemorrhage associated with renal failure
    - Anti-GBM Ab cross-reaction with pulmonary alveolar BM causes hemoptysis, hematuria, proteinuria and hypertension
  ○ The Goodpasture Ag
    - Unclear in most patients
    - Exposure to viruses or various drugs

类型2　快速进行性肾小球肾炎/急进性肾小球肾炎

概念

- 以肾小球囊壁层上皮细胞增生为特征,形成新月体

- 又称新月体性肾小球肾炎

发病机理与分类

- 大部分病例是由免疫机制引起的,根据病理学和免疫学可分为三种类型

- 抗肾小球基底膜抗体性肾小球肾炎
  ○ 免疫荧光
    - IgG、C3 的线性荧光
    - 抗GBM抗体与肺泡基膜发生交叉反应

  ○ 临床表现　肺出血肾炎综合征

    - 肺出血伴肾衰

    - 抗GBM抗体与肺泡基膜发生交叉反应,导致咯血,血尿,蛋白尿和高血压

  ○ 肺出血肾炎综合征抗原
    - 在大部分病人不清楚
    - 暴露在病毒和多种药物下

- Cigarette smoking
- Genetic predisposition to autoimmunity
- Immune-complex GN
  - Causes
    - Postinfectious GN development
    - Associated with systemic lupus erythematosus (SLE)
  - Electronic Microscopically
    - Electron-dense deposits of BM and mesangium
  - Immunofluorescence
    - Granular (BM, mesangium)
  - Features
    - Crescent formation immune complex
- Pauci-immune type
  - Electronic Microscopically or immunofluorescence
    - There are minimal immune deposits or none
  - Pathogenesis
    - Non-immune mechanism or Cell immunity
  - Antineutrophil cytoplasmic antibody (ACNA)
    - Always associated with some forms of vasculitis

Pathological changes
- Grossly
  - Kindey   enlarged, pale, Cortical

- 吸烟
- 自身免疫的遗传易感性
- 免疫复合物性肾小球肾炎
  - 病因
    - 感染后性肾小球肾炎发展而来
    - 与系统性红斑狼疮（SLE）相关
  - 电镜
    - 基膜和系膜有电子致密沉积物
  - 免疫荧光
    - 颗粒状（基底膜、系膜区）
  - 特征
    - 新月形免疫复合物形成
- 免疫反应缺乏性肾小球肾炎
  - 电镜和免疫荧光
    - 少量免疫沉积物或者没有
  - 发病机制
    - 非免疫机制或细胞免疫
  - 抗中性粒细胞胞质抗体（ACNA）
    - 总是与某些血管炎有关

病理变化
- 大体
  - 肾脏   增大、苍白、皮质增厚、可

petechial and Hemorrhage

- Microscopically
  - Glomerulus The formation of distinctive crescents; Proliferation of parietal cells; Infiltration of monocytes and macrophages; Because exudation of fibrin incites crescent formation
  - Crescents The early crescents mainly consisted of cellular components, called cellular crescents. After that, collagen fibers increased and transformed into fibrous-cellular crescent, eventually forming fibrous crescents
  - Renal tubules hyaline change Intracellular hyaline
  - Interstitium Edema and inflammatory cell infiltration
- Electronic Microscopically
  - Crescents
  - Distinct ruptures of GBM
- Immunofluorescence
  - Linear
  - Granular
  - No fluorescence

Clinical-Pathological Features

- Hematuria and proteinuria
  - Injury of the capillary wall (GBM) increases the permeability

见淤点及点状出血

- 镜下
  - 肾小球 新月体形成；壁细胞增生；单核细胞和巨噬细胞的浸润；纤维素生成促进新月体形成
  - 新月体 早期新月体以细胞成分为主，称为细胞性新月体，之后胶原纤维增多，转变为纤维—细胞性新月体，最终形成纤维性新月体
  - 肾小管玻璃样变 细胞内透明样变
  - 间质 水肿和炎细胞浸润
- 电镜
  - 可见新月体
  - 肾小球基底膜断裂
- 免疫荧光
  - 线性
  - 颗粒状
  - 无免疫荧光沉积物

临床病理特征

- 血尿或蛋白尿
  - 毛细血管壁（GBM）损伤会增加通透性，导致血尿和蛋白尿

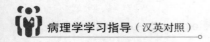

- Oliguria or anuria
  - Crescent formation obstructs Bowman's space, which compress the capillary tuft, So GFR↓↓
- Renal failure
  - Fibrosis and hyaline change of glomerulus cause loss of nephron function

Type 3　Membranous Glomerulonephritis

Conception

- Membranous Glomerulonephritis is an important and common cause of nephrotic syndrome in adults (mean age 35 years)
- Also known as membranous nephropathy

Etiology

- 85% idiopathic
- Autoantibody and complement

Pathological changes

- Grossly
  - Bilateral kidneys enlargement, pale in color
  - known as the large white kidney
- Microscopically
  - Diffuse thickening of glomerular capillary walls
- Electronic Microscopically
  - The epithelial cells were enlarged and the foot processes disappeared

- 少尿或无尿
  - 新月体阻塞了肾球囊，压迫肾小球毛细血管球，导致肾小球滤过率下降
- 肾功能衰竭
  - 肾小球纤维化和玻璃样变导致肾功能衰竭

类型3　膜性肾小球肾炎

概述

- 膜性肾小球肾炎是引起成年人肾病综合征最重要且普遍的原因（平均年龄35岁）

- 又称膜性肾病

病因

- 85%特发性
- 自身抗体和补体

病理变化

- 大体
  - 双肾肿大，颜色苍白

  - 有大白肾之称
- 光镜
  - 肾小球毛细血管壁弥漫性增厚

- 电镜
  - 上皮细胞肿胀，足突消失

- There were a large number of electron dense deposits between the basal membrane and the epithelium
- The basal membrane like substances increased and forming spiky processes between the deposits
- Immunofluorescence
  - IF shows granular deposits of IgG and C3 corresponding to the subepithelial deposits
- Clinical Features
  - Either the nephrotic syndrome or asymptomatic proteinuria
  - Most patients have a slow progression to chronic renal failure
  - The prognosis is better in females and much better in children

Type 4　Minimal Change Glomerulonephritis

Conception

- Most minimal change glomerulonephritis involving young children, rarely in adults
- It accounts for 80% of cases nephritic syndrome in children under 8 years old
- It is characterized by disappearance of epithelial cell foot process, so called foot process disease
- There are lipid deposits in epithelial cell of renal tubules, so called lipid nephropathy

- 基膜与上皮之间有大量电子致密沉积物
- 沉积物之间基膜样物质增多,形成钉状突起
- 免疫荧光
  - 免疫球蛋白IgG和C3补体呈颗粒状荧光沉积上皮下
- 临床特征
  - 肾病综合征,部分呈无症状蛋白尿
  - 大多数患者呈缓慢进展的慢性肾功能衰竭
  - 女性预后较好,儿童预后更好

类型4　微小病变性肾小球肾炎(足突病)

概述

- 微小病变性肾小球肾炎最常见于幼儿,在成年人中相对较少见
- 占8岁以下儿童肾病综合征病例的80%
- 以上皮细胞的足突消失为主要特征,又称足突病
- 肾小管上皮细胞内有脂质沉积,又称脂性肾病

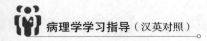

Etiology

- Minimal change GN is association with infections, immunizations
- Excellent response to immunosuppressive drugs such as corticosteroids
- Association with Hodgkin's lymphoma (where T lymphocyte abnormalities are common)
- T lymphomas from patients with minimal change GN produce lymphokines when cultured with kidney tissue, suggesting that minimal change GN may be a cell-mediated immune disease

Pathological change

- Microscopically   No abnormality (hence the term minimal change) in glomerulus. There are lipid deposits in epithelial cell of renal tubules
- Immunofluorescence   IF shows absence of immunoglobulin or complement deposition
- Electronic Microscopically   EM shows fusion of the foot processes of the epithelial cells (podocytes)

Clinical Feature

- Most nephritic syndrome in children
- Highly selective proteinuria, only loss of small anionic proteins
- Hematuria and hypertension are absent

Prognosis

- Most patients showing complete

病因学

- 微小病变性GN与感染、免疫相关
- 对皮质类固醇等免疫抑制药物反应良好
- 与霍奇金淋巴瘤相关（其中T淋巴细胞的异常很常见）
- 微小病变性GN患者的T淋巴瘤与肾脏组织一起培养时会产生淋巴因子，这表明微小病变性GN可能是一种细胞介导的免疫疾病

病理变化

- 光镜   肾小球无明显异常；肾小管上皮细胞内有脂质沉积
- 免疫荧光   显示无免疫球蛋白或补体沉积
- 电镜   显示上皮细胞（足突细胞）的足突融合

临床特征

- 儿童最常见的肾病综合征原因
- 高度选择性蛋白尿，仅损失小分子阴离子蛋白
- 无血尿，高血压

预后

- 大多数患者在8周内可完全缓解，

remission within 8 weeks. Corticosteroid therapy causes a dramatic decrease in proteinuria

- About 50% of patients relapse intermittently for up to 10 years after withdraw of steroids

Type 5   Focal Segmental Glomerulonephritis

Conception

- Segmental GN is an uncommon disease
- Accounts for 10% of cases of nephritic syndrome in children and young adults
- The cause is unknown

Pathological change

- Microscopically
  - Characterized by the presence of a focal segmental sclerotic area (aterial pink hyaline) in the peripheral part of the glomerulus, frequently near the hilum
  - Lipid droplets are often present as vacuoles in the sclerotic area
- Immunofluorescence
  - IF shows granular IgM, C3 and sometimes IgA, fibrinogen deposition in the affected glomeruli
- Electronic Microscopically
  - EM shows mesangial matrix increase and collapse of the glomerular capillaries in areas of

糖皮质激素治疗可导致蛋白尿急剧下降

- 类固醇停用后,约有50%的患者间歇性复发长达10年

类型5   局灶性节段性肾小球肾炎

概述

- 局灶性节段性GN是一种不常见的疾病
- 占儿童和年轻人肾病综合征病例的10%
- 原因尚不清楚

病理变化

- 光镜
  - 肾小球外围(通常在肾门附近)存在局灶性节段性硬化区(粉红色透明血管)
  - 硬化区常有脂滴
- 免疫荧光
  - IF显示在受影响的肾小球中IgM,C3,IgA和纤维蛋白原呈颗粒状沉积
- 电镜
  - EM示肾小球硬化区域肾小球毛细血管系膜基质增多和塌陷

glomerulosclerosis

○ Epithelial cell foot processes are fused

Clinical features

● It is associated with nephritic syndrome in children and adults

● It is poor with slow progression to chronic renal failure

Type 6　Membranoproliferative Glomerulonephritis

Conception

● Most membranoproliferative GN have no known cause

● Involving children and young adult

● It is characterized by deposition of subendothelial immune complexes in the glomerular capillary

Pathological change

● Microscopically

○ There has diffuse thickening of capillary basal membrane

○ Proliferation of mesangial cells and matrix

○ The inserted mesangial matrix and basement membrane appears to be split

○ Gomori's methenamine silver staining or PASM staining shows double-contour, or tram-track appearance

● Immunofluorescence

○ IF shows granular deposition of

○ 上皮细胞足突融合

临床特征

● 儿童和成人均表现为肾病综合征

● 预后不良,常缓慢进展为慢性肾功能衰竭

类型6　膜增生性肾小球肾炎

概述

● 大多数病例原因不明

● 主要见于儿童及年轻人

● 特点是肾小球毛细血管内皮下免疫复合物沉积

病理变化

● 光镜

○ 毛细血管基底膜弥漫性增厚

○ 肾小球系膜细胞及系膜基质增生

○ 系膜基质插入与基底膜形成特征性叶片状结构

○ 六胺银或PASM染色呈双线或双轨征

● 免疫荧光

○ 免疫荧光显示IgG和C3在毛细管

IgG and C3 in the capillary wall
- Electronic Microscopically
  - EM shows subendothelial deposits

Clinical Features

- Most of the cases are children and young adults who present with nephritic syndrome or a mixed nephritic-nephrotic pattern
- The overall prognosis is poor

Type 7   Mesangial proliferative Glomerulonephritis

Conception

- The pathogenesis is unknown in the most cases
- IgG deposition is common and may occur as an isolated finding or in the healing phase of post infectious glomerulonephritis

Pathological change

- Microscopically
  - The number of mesangial cells is increased in the glomeruli
  - The mesangial matrix material is increased
- Immunofluorescence
  - IF shows the presence of IgG or IgM and C3 in the mesangium
  - It is common IgM deposit in western country, so called IgM nephropathy

壁中呈颗粒状沉积
- 电镜
  - EM下显示毛细血管内皮下电子致密物沉积

临床特征

- 大多数儿童和青少年表现为肾病综合征或混合性肾炎性肾病综合征

- 总体预后差

类型7   系膜增生性肾小球肾炎

概述

- 大部分病例发病机制尚不清楚

- IgG沉积多见于部分感染后性肾小球肾炎的康复阶段

病理变化

- 光镜
  - 肾小球系膜细胞数量增加

  - 肾小球系膜基质增加

- 免疫荧光
  - 系膜出现IgG或IgM和C3

  - 西方多为IgM，又称IgM肾病

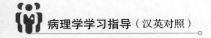

- Electronic Microscopically
  - EM shows the presence of mesangial electron-dense deposits in some cases

Clinical Features

- More common in children and young adults
- The symptom is associated with nephritic syndrome or asymptomatic proteinuria and/or hemaurine
- Prognosis is various, some good, but recurrent
- However, some poor, with slow progression to chronic renal failure

Type 8　IgA nephropathy

Conception

- The etiology of IgA nephropathy is unknown
- It accounts for 10% of cases of nephritic syndrome in both adults and children
- It is most common in the age group from 10 ～ 30 years old male predominant

Pathological change

- Microscopically
  - There is mesangial hypercellularity and increased matrix material
  - Sclerosis is common with progressive disease
- Immunofluorescence
  - IF show IgA deposits as confluent

- 电镜
  - 电镜下某些病例中出现系膜电子致密物沉积

临床特征

- 多见于儿童和年轻人
- 多表现为肾病综合征，或无症状蛋白尿和/或血尿
- 预后差异大，部分预后较好，但易复发
- 预后差者进展为慢性肾功能衰竭

类型8　IgA肾病

概念

- IgA肾病病因不明
- 占成年人和儿童肾病综合征病例的10%
- 最常见于10～30岁，男性为主

病理变化

- 光镜
  - 肾小球系膜细胞增多，系膜基质多
  - 进展期病例可见硬化
- 免疫荧光
  - IgA在系膜区沉积，呈融合块状或

masses or discrete granules in the mesangium
- C3 is frequently present
- Electronic Microscopically
  - EM shows mesangial hypercellularity, sclerosis, and electron-dense deposits

Clinical Features
- Patients present with hematuria, often at the time of an upper respiratory infection
- Hematuria is frequently recurrent
- Proteinuria and microscopic hematuria commonly persist
- The prognosis is not good though progression of the disease is very slow

Type 9   Chronic Glomerulonephritis

Conception
- It is a common pathologic lesion in the kidney that probably represents the end stage of many diseases affecting glomeruli
- Most patients give a past history suggestive of glomerular disease

Pathological change
- Grossly
  - The kidneys are greatly reduced in size, and the cortex shows a finely irregular surface (granular contracted kidney)
  - The cortex is narrowed, corticomedullary

散在颗粒

- 常伴有补体C3
- 电镜
  - 电镜显示肾小球系膜细胞增生，硬化和电子密集物沉积

临床特征
- 患者常在上呼吸道感染时出现血尿

- 反复发作的血尿
- 长期出现蛋白尿和镜下血尿

- 疾病进展缓慢，但预后不好

类型9   慢性肾小球肾炎

概述
- 慢性肾小球肾炎代表了许多肾小球疾病的终末阶段

- 大部分患者有肾小球疾病病史

病理变化
- 大体
  - 肾脏体积明显变小，肾表面不规则（颗粒固缩肾）

  - 肾皮质变窄，皮髓质界限模糊

demarcation is obscured

  ○ The arteries stand out because of thickened wall

○ 动脉因壁厚而突出

- Microscopically

  ○ The narrowed cortex shows a great decrease in the number of nephrons

  ○ Glomeruli show diffuse sclerosis, with many converted to hyaline balls

  ○ There is atrophy of intervening tubules

  ○ Residual tubules often show dilation and are filled with pink proteinaceous material

  ○ Interstitial fibrosis is present and severe

- 镜下

  ○ 肾皮质变窄，肾单位数量大大减少

  ○ 肾小球呈弥漫性硬化，许多肾小球玻璃样变

  ○ 肾小管萎缩

  ○ 残留的肾小管常扩张，并充满粉红色蛋白质物质

  ○ 肾间质纤维化明显

- IF and EM   show variable changes

  ○ Less fibrotic glomeruli may show evidence of electron-dense deposits containing IgG, IgA, and C3

  ○ These are important in distinguishing chronic GN from other conditions such as hypertensive nephrosclerosis and chronic pyelonephritis

- 免疫荧光和电镜   显示不同的改变

  ○ 纤维化轻的肾小球可能含有IgG，IgA和C3的电子致密沉积证据

  ○ 对区分慢性肾小球肾炎、高血压性肾硬化和慢性肾盂肾炎等疾病具有重要价值

Clinical features

- Patients show chronic renal failure and hypertension

- Some patients frequently have microscopic hematuria, proteinuria

- Sometimes nephrotic syndrome

临床特征

- 患者表现出慢性肾衰竭和高血压

- 常有镜下血尿，蛋白尿

- 有时出现肾病综合征

Summary of Glomerulonephritis

Types	lesion site	Hyperplastic cells	Pathological changes	Clinical features	Clinical manifestation	Pathological features
Acute GN	Intra-capillary	Mesangial cells Endothelial cells	Subendothelial cells,between subepithelial cells and GBM "Humps" electron-dense deposits	Children	Acute nephritic syndrome	Post infection of upper respiratory tract Enlarged red kidney flea-biting kidney
Crescentic GN	Extra-capillary	Parietal epithelial cells	Crescent formation	Good pasture syndrome	Rapidly progressive nephritic syndrome	Crescents
Membranous GN	Capillary wall	Capillary wall diffusely thickened	Basement membrane thickened Subepithelial deposits	Adult nephrotic syndrome	Nephrotic syndrome	Large white kidney
Minimal Change GN	Podocyte	Disappearance of epithelial cell foot process	Diffuse disappearance of epithelial cell foot process Lipid droplets in renal tubule epithelium	Child nephrotic syndrome	Nephrotic syndrome	Foot process disease lipid nephropathy
Segmental GN	Podocyte	Epithelial cell	Focally foot processes a fused	Adult and Children	Nephrotic syndrome	Focal lesion
Membranoproliferative GN	capillary basal membrane mesangial cells and matrix	Diffuse thickening of capillary basal membrane Proliferation of mesangial cells and matrix	Dual-track shape	Children and young adult	Nephrotic syndrome	Dual-track shape
Mesangial proliferative	Mesangial cells and matrix	Mesangial cells and matrix	Thicken of mesangial membrane	Adolescent teenager	Nephrotic syndrome	IgM diseases
Ig A nephropathy	mesangial membrane	Mesangial cells		Children and teenager	Recurrent hematuria	Post-infection
Chronic GN			Hyaline sclerosis of glomeruli		Renal failure	Terminal nephritis

肾小球肾炎总结

类　　型	病变部位	增生细胞	病理特征	临床特征	临床表现	特　　征
急性肾炎	毛细血管内	内皮细胞＋系膜细胞	脏层上皮细胞与GBM间驼峰样电子致密物沉积	小儿多见	急性肾炎综合征	上感后 大红肾 蚤咬肾
新月体肾炎	毛细血管外	壁层上皮细胞	新月体形成	肺出血肾炎综合征	急进性肾炎综合征	新月体
膜性肾炎	毛细血管壁	毛细血管壁弥漫性增厚	基底膜增厚 上皮下致密物	成人肾病综合征	肾病综合征	大白肾
微小病变	足突细胞	足突消失	弥漫性脏层上皮细胞足突消失 肾小管上皮内细胞脂滴	儿童肾病综合征	肾病综合征	足突病 脂性肾病
节段肾炎	足突细胞	脏层上皮细胞	局灶性足突融合	成人及儿童	肾病综合征	局灶性
膜性增生性肾炎	基底膜＋系膜细胞及基质	基底膜，系膜细胞与基质均增生	双轨状	儿童和青年	肾病综合征	双轨状
系膜增生性肾炎	系膜细胞及基质	系膜细胞及基质	系膜增厚	青少年	肾病综合征	IgM病
IgA肾病	系膜区	系膜区细胞可增生		儿童和青年	反复发作血尿	感染后
慢性肾炎			肾小球玻璃样变硬化		肾衰	终末肾炎

Section 2 Tubulointerstitial diseases

🖋 Conception of Pyelonephritis

- Pyelonephritis is inflammatory disease involving renal pelvis, and tubules interstitial tissue
- There are acute and chronic pyelonephritis

🖋 Acute Pyelonephritis

Conception

- It is extremely common, more often in females than in male (10 : 1)
- And it occurs at all ages, with highest frequency during pregnancy

Etiology

- A bacterial infection, usually ascending from the lower urinary tract
- Ascent of infection from the bladder is facilitated when vesicoureteral reflux is present
- Bacteria spread from the renal pelvis to the tubules by intrarenal reflux

Factors important in etiology

- A short urethra, as in females
- Stasis of urine from any cause
- Anatomy of urethra abnormalities
- Vesicoureteral reflux of urine
- Diabetes mellitus
- Seventy-five percent of cases of

第2节 肾小管肾间质疾病

🖋 肾盂肾炎概述

- 肾盂肾炎是肾盂、肾间质、肾小管的炎性病变
- 肾盂肾炎分急性和慢性

🖋 急性肾盂肾炎

概述

- 急性肾盂肾炎是一种非常普遍的疾病,女性多于男性(10 : 1)
- 可发生在任何年龄段,以怀孕期间发生率最高

病因学

- 细菌感染,通常从下泌尿道上行
- 膀胱输尿管反流易于增加膀胱感染
- 细菌通过肾内反流从肾盂扩散到肾小管

病因学中的重要因素

- 尿道短,如女性
- 因任何原因的尿液潴留
- 尿道结构异常
- 膀胱输尿管反流
- 糖尿病
- 75%的急性肾盂肾炎是由大肠埃希

acute pyelonephritis are causes by Escherichia coli

Pathological changes

- Grossly
  - Involving unilateral or bilateral
  - The kidney is enlarged and shows areas of suppuration (abscesses) in the cortex with radial yellow streaks traversing the medulla
- Microscopically
  - There is an acute suppurative inflammation beginning in the renal tubules, which show infiltration by neutrophils and hyperemia
  - Maybe following liquefactive necrosis of the tubules (suppuration)

Clinical Features

- Most cases present high fever, chills, rigors, and flank pain at onset
- Most patients present dysuria and frequency increased of urination
- The urine shows mild proteinuria, with neutrophils, white cell casts, and bacteria
- The prognosis is excellent. Most patients recover completely with treatment of antibiotics

Chronic Pyelonephritis

Conception

- Chronic Pyelonephritis accounts for

菌引起的

病理变化

- 大体
  - 累及单侧或双侧
  - 肾脏肿大，肾皮质可见脓液或脓肿，呈放射状黄色条纹横穿皮髓质

- 镜下
  - 肾小管开始出现急性化脓性炎症，表现为中性粒细胞浸润和充血

  - 肾小管液化性坏死（化脓性）

临床特征

- 起病时发高热，发冷，寒战和胁腹痛

- 多数情况下存在排尿困难和尿频

- 尿液显示轻度蛋白尿，中性粒细胞，白细胞管型和细菌

- 预后良好，大多数患者通过抗生素治疗可完全康复

慢性肾盂肾炎

概述

- 慢性肾盂肾炎占慢性肾衰竭病例的

15%～20% of cases of chronic renal failure

- Most patients have a history of a previous episode of acute pyelonephritis

- It can be divided into two types: Chronic obstructive pyelonephritis (calculi, prostatic hyperplasia, tumors); chronic pyelonephritis associated with vesicoureteral reflux

Pathological changes

- Grossly

  ○ Kidney show asymmetric involvement, with irregular scaring and contraction

  ○ Deep cortical pits due to scaring over a deformed renal calix are typical

  ○ Deformity of the pelvicaliceal system is common

  ○ Hydronephrosis and suppuration may be present in cases due to obstruction

- Microscopically

  ○ There is marked patchy inflammation and fibrosis of the interstitium of kidney

  ○ The inflammatory cells are lymphocytes and plasma cells with scattered neutrophils

  ○ Periglomerular fibrosis later progresses to global sclerosis

15%～20%

- 多数病人有急性肾盂肾炎发作史

- 可分为两种类型：慢性阻塞性肾盂肾炎（结石，前列腺增生，肿瘤）；伴有膀胱输尿管反流的慢性肾盂肾炎

病理变化

- 大体

  ○ 肾脏不对称受累，可见不规则的瘢痕和收缩

  ○ 肾盏变形、瘢痕形成导致肾皮质凹陷

  ○ 肾盂肾盏变形很常见

  ○ 因阻塞而导致肾积水和化脓性炎

- 镜下

  ○ 肾间质呈明显斑片状炎症和纤维化

  ○ 炎症细胞以淋巴细胞和浆细胞为主，可散在中性粒细胞

  ○ 肾小球硬化从肾小球周围开始，最终全部累及

○ Hypertrophy and dilation of surviving tubules may be present, maybe have casts in tubules, looks like thyroid follicle

Clinical Features

● Usually manifests as hypertension or chronic renal failure

● Pyuria (neutrophils in urine)

● Mild proteinuria, and bacteriuria are present

○ 残存肾小管肥大和扩张,可见管型,似甲状腺滤泡

临床特征

● 通常表现为高血压或慢性肾功能衰竭

● 常见脓尿（尿液出现中性粒细胞）

● 轻度蛋白尿和细菌尿

Section 3　Tumor of urinary system

第3节　泌尿系统肿瘤

Renal Cell Carcinoma (RCC)

Conception

● Renal cell carcinoma is the most common malignant neoplasm of the kidney

● Most frequently in the old adults, and Male : female = (2～3) : 1

● It is derived from tubular epithelial cells

Pathological changes

● Grossly

○ Location　Most RCC occurs in the up or down poles of the kidney

○ Shape　Most round, the margin is clear

○ Cut surface　Solid, maybe cystic

肾细胞癌

概述

● 肾细胞癌是肾脏最常见的恶性肿瘤

● 老年人最常见,男：女 = (2～3) : 1

● 大部分来源于肾小管上皮细胞

病理变化

● 大体

○ 部位　多数发生在肾脏的上下两极

○ 形状　多数圆形,界限清楚

○ 切面　通常实性,可以囊性,橙黄

with yellow-orange areas mottled with hemorrhagic and fibrous areas

- Microscopically
  ○ The most common RCC is clear cell renal carcinoma

Clinical Features and Prognosis

- RCC easily metastasizes to lungs or bones
- The 5 years survival less than 45%
- RCC can remain dormant stage for long periods, and cases have been recorded in which a metastatic lesion has occurred up to 30 years after treatment of the primary tumor

色的区域杂有出血和纤维化区域

- 镜下
  ○ 最常见的肾细胞癌是透明细胞肾癌

临床特征和预后

- 肾细胞癌经常转移至肺和骨

- 5年存活率＜45%
- 可以长期处于休眠状态,已有在治疗原发肿瘤后30年内发生转移性病变的病例

秦　铭　何妙侠

Chapter 11

Diseases of Genital System and Breast

Section 1　Diseases of cervix

🖋 Chronic cervicitis

Conception

- Chronic cervicitis is most commonly seen at the external cervix and endocervical canal
- This "exposed" columnar epithelium may appear reddened and moist and has been called cervical "erosion"

Pathological changes

- Grossly
  - Squamous metaplasia of the endocervical epithelium is common, probably representing a response to irritation
  - Polyps are common lesions of the endocervical canal, usually occurring at about the time of menopause. When large, a polyp

第 11 章

生殖系统与乳腺疾病

第 1 节　宫颈疾病

🖋 慢性宫颈炎

概述

- 慢性宫颈炎最常见于宫颈外口和宫颈管

- "暴露的"柱状上皮可能呈现红色和潮湿，被称为宫颈"糜烂"

病理变化

- 大体
  - 宫颈上皮的鳞状上皮化生很常见，可能是对刺激的反应

  - 息肉是宫颈管的常见病变，通常发生于绝经前后。当息肉变大时易突出子宫颈外口

may protrude out of the external cervix

- Microscopically
  - Moderate numbers of lymphocytes, plasma cells, and histiocytes are present in the cervix in all females
  - Chronic cervicitis is therefore difficult to define pathologically

Cervix Squamous Dysplasia

- Dysplasia commonly involves the region of the squamo-columnar junction and the endocervical canal that has undergone squamous metaplasia
- Dysplasia is recognized by the presence of cytologic abnormalities in a cervical smear and confirmed by cervical biopsy
- Nowadays, we use the terminology of squamous intraepithelial lesion (SIL) for squamous dysplasia, it can be classified two grade including low and high grade (LSIL and HSIL)

Squamous Carcinoma of the Cervix

Conception

- Squamous carcinoma of the Cervix is the most frequent form of cancer in women around the world once
- It is associated with HPV infection, particularly HPV16 and 18

- 镜下
  - 所有女性子宫颈中均可见中等量淋巴细胞、浆细胞和组织细胞
  - 慢性宫颈炎很难从病理学上定义

宫颈上皮不典型增生

- 异型增生通常发生在鳞状上皮与柱状上皮交界处和宫颈管上皮鳞状上皮化生的基础上
- 异型增生可通过子宫颈涂片上的细胞学异常和宫颈活检来确认
- 目前,我们使用鳞状上皮内病变(SIL)这一术语来描述鳞状上皮不典型增生,可分为低级别和高级别(LSIL和HSIL)

子宫颈鳞状细胞癌

概述

- 子宫颈鳞状细胞癌曾经是世界上女性最常见的癌症
- 与HPV感染有关,尤其是HPV16、18型感染有关

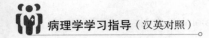

Pathological changes

- Grossly
  - It presents as an exophytic, fungating, necrotic mass or a malignant ulcer, or as a diffusely infiltrative lesion with only minimal surface ulceration or nodularity
- Microscopically   There are three different types
  - Keratinizing squamous carcinoma
  - Nonsquamous carcinoma
  - Adenocarcinoma

Section 2　Diseases of prostate

Benign prostatic hyperplasia

Also called benign nodular hyperplasia

- Grossly
  - The periurethral part of the prostate is most commonly involved because this area is sensitive to the estrogen
  - Overall, the prostate is enlarged, with a firm consistency
  - The cut surface shows multiple circumscribed solid nodules with small cysts
- Microscopically
  - The nodules are composed of a

病理变化

- 大体
  - 表现为外生型、菜花样、肿块或溃疡伴坏死，或弥漫性浸润性病变，只有表面溃疡或结节

- 镜下　有三种不同的类型

  - 角化型鳞状细胞癌
  - 非角化型鳞状细胞癌
  - 腺癌

第2节　前列腺疾病

良性前列腺增生

又称良性结节状增生

- 大体
  - 前列腺尿道部是最常受累，该处对雌激素很敏感

  - 总之前列腺变大、变实

  - 切面可见多个界限清楚的实性结节和囊肿

- 镜下
  - 结节由增生性腺体和纤维肌间质

variable mixture of hyperplastic glandular elements and hyperplastic fibromuscular stroma

○ The prostate is larger than normal and lined by tall epithelium that is frequently with papillary projections

组成

○ 腺体比正常的大，排列着高大的上皮，通常有乳头状突起

🖋 Prostate carcinoma

- The most common prostate carcinoma is acinar adenocarcinoma
- The tumor score is evaluated by Gleason score system

🖋 前列腺癌

- 最常见的前列腺癌是前列腺腺泡腺癌
- 肿瘤评分采用Gleason评分系统

Section 3 Diseases of breast

第3节 乳腺疾病

🖋 Breast Adenosis

- Breast Adenosis is a benign lesion in which the normal breast structure of the lobules is lost due to hyperplasia of mammary gland tissue
- It is characterized by different degrees of focal hyperplasia of acinar and ductules of the breast, usually with interstitial connective tissue hyperplasia

🖋 乳腺腺病

- 乳腺腺病是乳腺组织增生导致乳腺小叶正常结构消失的一种良性病变

- 表现为乳腺的腺泡和小导管明显的局灶性增生，并有不同程度间质结缔组织增生

🖋 Sclerosing Adenosis

- This variant is characterized by marked intralobular fibrosis and

🖋 硬化性乳腺病

- 这种乳腺腺病的特征是小叶内明显纤维化和腺泡增生伴变形及受压

increased number of distorted and compressed acini

Neoplasms of the Breast

Fibroadenoma of the Breast

- It presents as a discrete, firm, freely movable nodule in the breast
- Grossly
  ○ Fibroadenomas are encapsulated, firm, and uniformly grayish-white, 1～5 cm in diameter but may be larger
- Microscopically
  ○ Fibroadenomas are composed of both glandular and fibrous elements
  ○ The glands may be surrounded by stromal fibrosis or compressed and distorted

Carcinoma of The Breast

- The majority of breast cancer comes from the ductal epithelial and acinar epithelial dysplasia in the breast lobules
- Patients with invasive carcinoma always found breast mass, the breast skin is not easily movable or has an orange peel appearance

Lobular carcinoma in situ

- The lobules involved show acinar epithelial dysplasia filling terminal ductal lobular units and not yet

乳腺肿瘤

乳腺纤维腺瘤

- 纤维腺瘤在乳腺表现为界限清楚,质地偏硬,容易推动的结节
- 大体
  ○ 纤维腺瘤常有包膜,质地偏硬,呈均匀灰白色,直径1～5厘米或更大
- 镜下
  ○ 由腺体和纤维样间质组成腺体会被纤维间质挤压扭曲
  ○ 乳腺腺体被纤维化的间质包绕、挤压及扭曲

乳腺癌

- 乳腺癌多数来源于乳腺小叶内的导管上皮和腺泡上皮异型增生所致,其中大部分为乳腺导管上皮来源的肿瘤,分原位癌和浸润性癌
- 浸润性癌患者常有乳腺肿块,乳腺表面皮肤常固定或有橘皮样改变

小叶原位癌

- 所涉及的小叶显示腺泡上皮异型增生充填于终末导管小叶单位

- Infiltrate into the surrounding stroma

Ductal carcinoma in situ

- The tumor characterized by increased atypical proliferation of ductal epithelial cells confined within the intraductal area
- It has not yet infiltrated into the extraductal stroma

Invasive ductal carcinoma

- Grossly
  - Invasive carcinoma shows gray white irregular, qualitative hard mass
- Microscopically
  - The ductal epithelial cells of dysplasia infiltrate the ductal surrounding tissue

Therapy of breast cancer

- Breast cancer is mostly related to estrogen and may also be related to *HER2* gene amplification
- Therefore, detection of *ER* and *HER2* expression or *HER2* gene amplification can be used as the basis for anti-hormone therapy and anti-*HER2*-targeted therapy

- 尚未浸润到周围间质

导管原位癌

- 所涉及的导管内上皮细胞异型增生充填于导管内

- 尚未浸润到导管外的间质

浸润性导管癌

- 大体
  - 浸润性癌呈灰白色不规则、质硬肿块

- 镜下
  - 异型增生的导管上皮细胞浸润导管周围组织

乳腺癌治疗

- 乳腺癌多数与雌激素有关,也可能与*HER2*基因扩增有关

- 所以通过检测*ER*和*HER2*的表达或*HER2*基因扩增,可以作为抗激素治疗和抗*HER2*靶向治疗的依据

李满平　何妙侠

Chapter 12

Diseases of Endocrine System

Section 1　Diseases of the thyroid gland

🪶 Conception

- The endocrine system consists of pituitary, thyroid gland, pancreatic island and adrenal gland
- We are here introducing the diseases of thyroid gland and pancreatic island
- The thyroid gland consists of two bulky lateral lobes connected by a relatively thin isthmus, usually located below and anterior to the larynx
- The thyroid gland develops embryologically from an evagination of the developing pharyngeal epithelium that descends from the foramen cecum at the base of the tongue to its normal position in the anterior neck
- This pattern of the descent explains the occasional presence of ectopic

第 12 章

内分泌系统疾病

第 1 节　甲状腺疾病

🪶 概述

- 内分泌系统器官包括垂体、甲状腺、胰岛和肾上腺

- 我们在本章只介绍甲状腺和胰岛疾病
- 甲状腺由两个较大的侧叶组成，由相对较薄的峡部连接，位于喉下前方

- 甲状腺由咽部上皮发育而来，从舌根的盲孔下降到前颈

- 异位甲状腺组织是由于甲状腺胚胎发育异常所致，最常见于舌根（舌状

thyroid tissue, most commonly located at the base of the tongue (lingual thyroid) or at other sites abnormally high in the neck

甲状腺）或颈部其他部位

Goiter

Diffuse Nontoxic Goiter

Conception

- This goiter represents the culmination of mild deficiency of thyroid hormone production of followed by compensatory thyroid hyperplasia
- Serum TSH levels are normal
- Some cases are because of iodine deficiency, It is thought likely that there is an increased responsiveness of thyroid cells to TSH due to depletion of organic iodine in the cells resulting from impaired hormone synthesis
- Also called nodular goiter

Etiology

- The basic cause of the goiter is failure of normal thyroid hormone synthesis
- **Endemic Goiter** The result of chronic dietary deficiency of iodine in special regions
- **Sporadic Goiter** May occur anywhere and is usually due to increased physiologic demand for thyroxin
- Abnormalities relating to synthesis of

甲状腺肿

弥漫性非毒性甲状腺肿

概述

- 代表甲状腺激素产生的轻度缺乏以及随后的代偿性甲状腺的过度增生

- 血清TSH水平正常
- 部分缺碘，可能是由于激素合成过程受损导致细胞中有机碘耗竭，甲状腺细胞对TSH的分泌反应性的增加

- 又称结节性甲状腺肿

病因

- 甲状腺肿的根本原因是甲状腺激素合成不正常
- **流行性甲状腺肿** 特定地区长期饮食中缺乏碘

- **散发性甲状腺肿** 任何地方都可能发生，通常是由于对甲状腺素的生理需求增加所致

- 与甲状腺结合球蛋白合成异常有

thyroid-binding globulin may cause goiter because excess thyroxine-binding globulin in plasma decreases delivery of free hormone to the periphery

关,因为血浆中过量的甲状腺素结合球蛋白会减少游离激素向外周的输送

Pathological changes

- Grossly
  - It can be divided into hyperplasia stage, gelatinous storage stage and nodular stage according to the development process
  - Diffuse enlargement to multi-nodular appearance
  - The cut surface appears gelatinous and glistening owing to its colloid content
- Microscopically
  - The follicles become distended with colloid
  - The lining epithelial cells become flattened or cuboidal

Clinical Features

- Painless diffuse enlargement of the thyroid
- In a few patients, the presence of a dominant nodule may mimic a neoplastic process
- Abnormal thyroid hormone production may rarely occur in multinodular goiter
- The risk of development of carcinoma

病理变化

- 大体
  - 根据发生发展进程可分为增生期、胶质贮积期和结节期
  - 甲状腺弥漫性肿大或呈多结节状
  - 切面因含有胶质呈胶冻状
- 镜下
  - 甲状腺滤泡充满胶质而扩张
  - 滤泡上皮细胞扁平或呈立方状

临床特征

- 甲状腺无痛性弥漫性肿大
- 少数患者出现类似于肿瘤的结节
- 多结节性甲状腺肿很少出现甲状腺激素异常
- 多结节性甲状腺肿很少癌变

in a multinodular goiter is small

Diffuse Toxic Goiter (Hyperthyroidism)

Conception

- Diffuse Toxic Goiter is easily involvement the group of 15 to 40 years old patients
- Female more than male

Etiology

- An autoimmune disease characterized by the presence in serum of autoantibodies of the IgG class directed against the TSH receptors in the thyroid cells
- The combination of the antibody with the receptors leads to stimulating the cells to produce thyroid hormone

Pathological changes

- Grossly
  - Diffusely and symmetrically thyroid enlarged, especially vessels hyperemia
- Microscopically
  - Thyroid follicular epithelial cells are increased in size and number
  - The follicles are closely packed and lined by tall columnar epithelium which is frequently thrown into papillary infoldings
  - Colloid is scanty, and its periphery is scalloped
  - Lymphocytic infiltration of the

弥漫性毒性甲状腺肿（甲亢）

概述

- 弥漫性毒性甲状腺肿多发于15～40岁人群

- 女性多于男性

病因

- 属于自身免疫性疾病，其特征在于血清中存在针对甲状腺TSH受体的IgG类自身抗体

- 抗体与TSH受体结合可刺激甲状腺产生甲状腺激素

病理变化

- 大体
  - 甲状腺弥漫性、对称性肿大，尤其是血管充血明显

- 镜下
  - 甲状腺滤泡上皮细胞增生、变大

  - 甲状腺滤泡排列拥挤，滤泡上皮呈高柱状，呈乳头状褶皱

  - 滤泡腔内胶质稀薄，外围可见吸收空泡
  - 间质较多淋巴细胞浸润，可见淋

interstitium is common, and lymphoid follicles with germinal centers may be present

巴滤泡形成，并出现生发中心

Clinical Features

- Diffuse enlarged and appears as a mass in the neck

- The greatly increased blood flow is often present over the gland

- Eye changes (exophthalmos) the external muscle edema of eyeballs. There are connective tissue hyperplasia, lymphocyte infiltrate and myxedema behind the eyeball

- Laboratory evidence of hyperthyroidism-most reliably elevation of free thyroxine T3 and T4 index is present

临床特征

- 弥漫性肿大并在颈部出现肿块

- 甲状腺血流量大大增加

- **眼球突出** 原因是眼球外肌水肿，球后结缔组织增生、淋巴细胞浸润和黏液水肿

- 甲亢最可靠的诊断指标为血清游离甲状腺素 T3 和 T4 升高

Thyroiditis

Subacute thyroiditis

Conception

- Also called subacute granulomatous thyroiditis
- Belong to virus infectious thyroiditis
- Mainly involving young female
- The patient has an acute onset and may have fever

Pathological changes

- Grossly Thyroid enlarged with nodularity, the cut surface showed scar
- Microscopically There are focal lesions, some thyroid follicle destructed,

甲状腺炎

亚急性甲状腺炎

概述

- 又叫亚急性肉芽肿性甲状腺炎

- 属于病毒感染性甲状腺炎
- 主要累及中青年女性
- 病人起病急，可有发热

病理变化

- **大体** 甲状腺呈结节状增大，切面可有瘢痕
- **镜下** 病变呈多灶性 一些甲状腺滤泡破坏，形成类似结核、结节的肺

forming granulomas that resemble tuberculosis nodules

- There are many Foreign body giant cells, but without caseous necrosis
- There are inflammatory cells such as neutrophils, eosinophils, lymphocytes and plasma cell

Chronic lymphocytic thyroiditis
Conception

- Also called Hashimoto's thyroiditis
- Belong to autoimmune thyroiditis
- Involving middle-aged female
- There are autoimmune antibodies
- Serum free thyroxine T3and T4 decreased, and TSH is increased

Pathological changes

- Grossly   Thyroid diffuse enlarged
- Microscopically   Thyroid follicle epithelial cell injury and acidophilic change, lymphocyte hyperplasia and form lymph follicle, fibrotic tissue proliferation in the interstitial tissue

Prognosis

- Some patients develop tumor, including papillary carcinoma or lymphoma

Thyroid Neoplasms
Thyroid adenoma
Conception

- Thyroid adenoma is common neoplasm of the thyroid, accounting for about

肉芽肿

- 可见外来巨细胞,但无干酪样坏死

- 可有炎细胞如中性粒细胞、嗜酸性粒细胞、淋巴细胞和浆细胞等浸润

慢性淋巴细胞性甲状腺炎
概述

- 又称桥本甲状腺炎
- 属于自身免疫性甲状腺炎
- 常累及中年女性
- 可有多种自身免疫抗体
- 血清游离甲状腺素 T3、T4 降低,TSH 升高

病理变化

- **大体**   甲状腺弥漫性肿大
- **镜下**   甲状腺滤泡上皮细胞损伤,嗜酸性变,淋巴细胞增生并形成淋巴滤泡,间质纤维化组织增生

预后

- 一些病人会发展为肿瘤,包括甲状腺乳头状癌或淋巴瘤

甲状腺肿瘤
甲状腺腺瘤
概述

- 甲状腺腺瘤为甲状腺常见肿瘤,约占所有孤立性甲状腺结节病例的30%

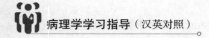

30% of all cases of solitary thyroid nodules

- It may occur at any age, but female is affected four times than males

Pathological feature

- Grossly
  - Solitary, firm gray or red nodular up to 5 cm in diameter
  - Hemorrhage, fibrosis, calcification, and cystic degeneration may be present
- Microscopically
  - This follicular adenoma always has capsule, as sole nodule
  - The morphology of tumor inside of nodule is different from outside, the normal thyroid parenchyma around the adenoma is compressed
  - The cytological features of follicles are uniform in inside of nodule
  - There is absence of capsule and vascular invasion

Clinical Features

- The thyroid usually enlargement
- Thyroid scan shows the presence of a circumscribed "cold" nodule

Thyroid carcinoma

Conception

- The incidence of thyroid carcinoma has increased greatly in the last 50

可发生在任何年龄,但女性发病率是男性的4倍

病理特征

- 大体
  - 孤立,质硬的灰色或红色结节,直径≤5厘米
  - 可出现出血,纤维化,钙化和囊性变

- 镜下
  - 滤泡性腺瘤常有包膜,呈单个结节
  - 结节内的形态学特征与结节外不同,结节周围正常甲状腺组织受压迫

  - 结节内由滤泡及滤泡上皮细胞较一致的
  - 没有包膜和血管侵犯

临床特征

- 甲状腺肿大
- 甲状腺扫描显示境界清楚的"冷"结节

甲状腺癌

概述

- 甲状腺癌的发病率在过去50年来明显上升

years
- There are three types of thyroid carcinoma from thyroid follicular epithelium: papillary, follicular, and anaplastic carcinoma
- The most common type is papillary carcinoma
- Medullary carcinoma is distinct and arises in the para-follicular secreting calcitonin cells

Papillary carcinoma

Pathological features

- Thyroid papillary carcinoma is characterized by arrangement of cells in papillary structures, ground glass like nuclei, prominent nuclear grooves and intranuclear inclusions

Prognosis

- Papillary carcinomas grow slowly and it has a good prognosis after surgical resection
- Microcarcinoma or occult carcinoma refers to tumors with a diameter less than 1 cm with a better prognosis, but now we don't recommend to use this term
- They commonly spread by local invasion, and many have invaded the thyroid capsule at the time of presentation
- Lymphatic metastasis is common

- 来自甲状腺滤泡上皮的甲状腺癌包括乳头状癌、滤泡癌和间变性癌3种

- 最常见的类型是甲状腺乳头状癌

- 髓样癌来自于滤泡旁分泌降钙素的细胞

乳头状癌

病理特征

- 甲状腺乳头状癌的肿瘤细胞呈分枝乳头状排列，肿瘤细胞核呈毛玻璃样，排列拥挤，可见核沟和核内包涵体

预后

- 甲状腺乳头状癌生长缓慢，手术切除预后较好

- 微小癌或隐匿癌指直径＜1厘米的肿瘤，预后更好，但是现在不提倡使用这一术语

- 肿瘤通常通过局部浸润而播散，许多病例在诊断时已侵犯包膜

- 多通过淋巴道转移

Section 2　Diseases of the pancreatic islet

🍃 Diabetes Mellitus

Conception

- Diabetes Mellitus is a chronic disease characterized by relative or absolute deficiency of insulin, resulting in glucose intolerance

Etiology and types

- Diabetes Mellitus is caused by a relative or absolute deficiency of insulin
- The classic symptoms of diabetes mellitus result from abnormal glucose metabolism
- Primary diabetes has two types
  - Type Ⅰ Insulin-dependent diabetes mellitus, IDDM
  - Type Ⅱ Non-insulin-dependent diabetes mellitus (NIDDM)

Pathological feature

- Pancreatic islets lesions　The pathologic changes in the pancreatic islets are variable
  - In type I diabetes, there is frequently a lymphocytic infiltration in islets in the early stage, following by a progressive loss of β cells
  - The changes in type Ⅱ diabetes are often minimal in the early stages.

第2节　胰岛疾病

🍃 糖尿病

概念

- 以胰岛素相对或绝对缺乏为特征的慢性疾病,导致葡萄糖耐受不良

病因与类型

- 由于胰岛素相对或绝对不足引起

- 糖尿病的典型症状是葡萄糖代谢异常

- 原发性糖尿病有两种类型
  - 1型糖尿病　胰岛素依赖的糖尿病
  - 2型糖尿病　非胰岛素依赖的糖尿病（NIDDM）

病理特征

- 胰岛病变　病理变化多种多样

  - 1型糖尿病中,早期胰岛有淋巴细胞浸润,然后逐渐出现β细胞减少直至消失

  - 2型糖尿病中,早期变化很小,晚期胰岛纤维化和淀粉样物质沉积

In advanced stage, there may be fibrosis and amyloid deposition in the islets

- Small vessel lesions
  ○ Small vessel disease is one of the most characteristic and most important pathologic changes
  ○ It is characterized by diffuse thickening of the basement membranes of capillaries throughout the body
  ○ The small vessels of kidney, retina, skin, and skeletal muscles are commonly involved
- Large vessel disease
  ○ A major risk factor for development of atherosclerotic vascular disease
  ○ Myocardial infarction and cerebral arterial occlusion represent two of the most common causes of death in diabetics
  ○ Diabetic nephropathy nodular or diffuse glomerulosclerosis—Kimmelstiel-Wilson disease

Clinical Features

- Quality of life is seriously affected for all diabetics because of many disabling complications
- Causes of death in diabetes are myocardial infarction, renal failure, cerebrovascular accidents, infections

- 小血管疾病
  ○ 小血管病变是最典型,最重要的病理变化之一
  ○ 以全身毛细血管基底膜弥漫性增厚为特征
  ○ 常累及肾脏、视网膜、皮肤和骨骼肌小血管
- 大血管病变
  ○ 动脉粥样硬化性血管疾病发展的主要危险因素
  ○ 心肌梗死和脑动脉栓塞是糖尿病患者最常见的两种死亡原因
  ○ 糖尿病肾病,结节性或弥漫性肾小球硬化——基-威病

临床特征

- 由于血管病变导致的许多致残并发症,所有糖尿病患者的生活质量均都受到严重影响
- 糖尿病的死亡原因是心肌梗死,肾功能衰竭,脑血管意外,感染和低血糖

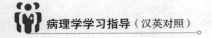
and hypoglycemia

- The average life expectancy of diabetics is reduced by 9 years for males and 7 years for females when compared with non-diabetics

- 与非糖尿病患者相比，男性糖尿病患者的平均预期寿命降低了9年，女性降低了7年

何　晨　何妙侠

Chapter 13

Infectious Diseases

Conception

- Infectious diseases are a group of diseases that can be transmitted by infectious sources in the population or between individuals

Characteristics of infectious diseases

- Although the features of pathologic change of infectious diseases are different, the basic pathologic changes are the same and belong to the inflammation
- The acute infectious disease is fibrous or purulent inflammation, such as bacillary dysentery or purulent meningitis
- Most chronic infectious disease are granulomatous inflammation such as Tuberculosis (TB), Syphilis and Typhoid

第 13 章

感染性疾病（传染病）

概述

- 传染病是传染源在人群中或个体间传播的一组感染性疾病

传染病的特点

- 尽管传染病的病理变化特征是不同的，但其基本病理改变是一样的，均属于炎症

- 急性传染病是纤维素性炎或化脓性炎，如细菌性痢疾和化脓性脑膜炎

- 大部分慢性传染病是肉芽肿性炎症，如结核、伤寒和梅毒

Basic factors of infectious diseases

- Infectious source
- Route of transmission
- Susceptible population

传染病的基本环节

- 传染源
- 传播途径
- 易感人群

Section 1　Tuberculosis, TB

第1节　结核病

Conception

- Tuberculosis (TB) is a chronic granulomatous disease caused by tubercle bacilli. The lung is the prime target, but any organ could be infected
- The Characteristic lesion of TB are the formation of tubercle and central caseous necrosis

概述

- 结核病是由结核分枝杆菌引起的慢性肉芽肿性疾病，好发于肺，其他任何器官均可以被感染

- 结核特征性病变是结核结节形成和中央干酪样坏死

Types of TB

- Pulmonary TB
  - Primary pulmonary TB
  - Secondary pulmonary TB
- Extra pulmonary TB
  - Intestinal TB
  - Tuberculous meningitis
  - Tuberculous peritonitis
  - TB of bone and joint
  - TB of lymph node
  - TB of urinary and genital system

结核病类型

- 肺结核
  - 原发性肺结核
  - 继发性肺结核
- 肺外结核
  - 肠结核
  - 结核性脑膜炎
  - 结核性腹膜炎
  - 骨关节结核
  - 淋巴结核
  - 泌尿生殖系统结核

Etiology and Pathogenesis of TB

- Routes of Transmission
  - Respiratory tract a main route to transmit, person to person direct transmission by sneeze, cough droplets with organisms (1 ～ 20 bacteria/droplet)
  - Digestive tract contaminated milk by bovine type
  - Local skin lesion rarely
- Pathogenic organism
  - Mycobacterium of tuberculosis (Gram positive), also called tuberculosis bacillus
  - Type Human and bovine types are pathogenic to humans; mouse and fish types are non-pathogenic to humans
- Pathogenic substance of tuberculosis bacillus
  - Lipid Related to pathogenicity. Especially, glycolipid factors damage the membrane of mitochondria and inhibit the migration of leukocytes and the formation of granuloma
  - Wax D Causes severe allergic reactions and tissue damage, inhibits bacterial fusing to lysosomes, protects bacteria from digestion by macrophages and allows bacteria

病因与发病机制

- 传播途径
  - 呼吸道 最主要的途径，人与人之间直接通过打喷嚏，带有细菌的飞沫（1 ～ 20 个细菌/飞沫）
  - 消化道 较少，被牛型结核分枝杆菌污染的牛奶
  - 皮肤 少见
- 病原微生物
  - 结核分枝杆菌（革兰阳性菌）
  - 类型 人型和牛型对人类致病；鼠、鱼型对人无致病性
- 结核分枝杆菌的致病物质
  - 脂质 与致病性有关，尤其是糖脂类因子破坏线粒体膜，抑制白细胞迁移及肉芽肿形成
  - 蜡质D 引起严重的过敏反应和组织损伤，抑制细菌与溶酶体的结合保护细菌免受巨噬细胞的消化，使细菌可以生存，磷脂将巨噬细胞转变为上皮样细胞

to survive. Phospholipids convert macrophages into epithelioid cells

- Polysaccharide lipoarabinomannan Inhibit the activity of macrophages and promote the secretion of TNF-α and IL-10 leading necrosis and inhibiting cell immune, respectively
- Complement Promoting phagocytosis
- Protein heat-shock protein, autoimmune reaction

- Pathogenesis
  - The Pathogenesis of tuberculosis Cellular immunity and Type IV hypersensitivity
  - There are three considerations involved in the pathogenesis of TB quantity of bacteria, Virulence of pathogen, Pathogenic bacteria toxic sensitization and immune response of the body

- Basic pathological changes of TB
  - Three basic pathological changes, inflammation, exudation and proliferation, can coexist or transform into each other in tuberculosis

- Early stage Mainly exudation
  - Conditions Immunity weak, the body's immunity is low, the number of bacteria is large, and the bacterial toxicity are strong

多糖脂质阿拉伯甘露聚糖 抑制巨噬细胞的活性,分泌TNF-α引起坏死,分泌IL-10抑制细胞免疫

补体 促进吞噬作用

蛋白 热休克蛋白,引起自身免疫反应

- 致病机制
  - 结核病的发病机制包括细胞免疫和IV型超敏反应

  - 致病过程涉及以下三方面因素:细菌的数量,细菌的毒力,致病菌的毒性,机体致敏性和免疫应答

- 结核基本病理变化
  - 炎症的变质、渗出和增生三大基本病理变化在结核中可同时存在或相互转化

- 早期 渗出性炎为主
  - 条件 早期机体免疫力低下,细菌数量多,细菌毒性强,引起严重的超敏反应

in the early stage, causing severe hypersensitivity reactions

○ **Pathologic changes** Serous or serofibrinous; excudation of neutrophils in early and macrophages in late

○ **Location** Lung, serosa, synovialis, meninges etc.

○ **Result** Absorbed completely, development proliferation or necrosis

● **Late stage** Mainly proliferative inflammation

○ **Conditions** In the later stage, the immunity of the body is enhanced. The number and toxicity of bacteria are reduced. The cellular immune response becomes the mainstay

○ **Pathologic changes** Formation of tubercle (diagnostic evidence)

○ **Grossly** Millet or small grayish, semi-transparent nodules with clear edge on the surface of the organ. Sometimes has yellowish necrosis

○ **Morphologically**
Formation of Tubercle (Based on cell immune) and necrosis

● **Typical tuberculosis granuloma**

○ **Center** Caseous necrosis

○ **Surrounding** Epithelioid cell and Langhans giant cell

○ **Outside** Lymphocyte and fibroblast

○ **病理变化** 纤维素或纤维蛋白；早期中性粒细胞渗出，后期巨噬细胞渗出

○ **发病部位** 肺，浆膜，滑膜，脑膜等

○ **结局** 大部分完全吸收，部分伴增生及坏死。

● **后期** 增生性炎症为主

○ **条件** 后期机体免疫力增强，细菌数量减少，细菌毒性下降，以免疫反应为主

○ **病理变化** 形成典型结核结节的形成（具有诊断意义）

○ **大体** 米粒大小、灰色、半透明边界清晰的结节，位于器官表面，黄色坏死

○ **镜下** 典型结核结节及干酪样坏死

● **典型结核肉芽肿**

○ **中央** 为干酪样坏死

○ **外围** 可见上皮样细胞和朗汉斯巨细胞

○ **周边** 淋巴细胞及成纤维细胞

- Epithelioid cells
  - Source   Macrophage
  - Shape   Large, abundant cytoplasm
  - Function   Phagocytize, Kill mycobacterium
- Langhans giant cell
  - Source   Fusion of epithelioid cells, division of nuclei without cytoplastic division
  - Shape   multi-nuclei, floral hoop or horseshoe-like, abundant cytoplasm
  - Function   Phagocytizing and killing mycobacterium
- Necrosis
  - Conditions   Immunity weak or resistance to therapy, high quantity of bacteria, strong virulence of bacteria, lead to severe allergy
  - Lesion   Caseous necrosis
  - Grossly   Slight yellow, homogenous, like exquisite creamy
  - Microscopically   Red staining, no structure, granular substance
  - Result   Not easily absorbed and autolyzed. Sometimes, they could be softened, liquefied, or calcified

Consequences of TB
- Completely healing
  - Healing or repairing
    - The main approach of cure is the extravasation through lymphatic

- 上皮样细胞
  - 来源   巨噬细胞
  - 形态   细胞大,胞质丰富
  - 功能   有一定吞噬能力,杀死结核杆菌
- 朗汉斯巨细胞
  - 来源   上皮样细胞融合,细胞质融合,细胞核没有融合

  - 形态   多核,呈花环或马蹄形,胞质丰富
  - 功能   吞噬,杀灭结核杆菌

- 坏死
  - 条件   机体免疫力下降或耐药,细菌数量多,细菌毒性强,引起严重的过敏反应

  - 病理变化   干酪样坏死
  - 大体   坏死呈淡黄色,均匀,细腻的奶酪状
  - 镜下   坏死呈红染,无结构的颗粒状物质
  - 结局   不易吸收,不自溶。有时会软化,液化或钙化

结核的转归
- 转向愈合
  - 治愈或修复
    - 通过淋巴管渗出的主要治愈方法

vessels

- Absorption and disappearance of small-scale necrosis

- Imaging The proliferative edge is not clear, dense and uneven cloud-like shadow

- Clinically need treatment, take measures

○ Fibrous encapsulation and calcification

- Fibrous encapsulation Proliferative nodules, exudates and fibrous cysts of small organized necrotic foci

- Calcification Large necrotic foci are calcified, dried, concentrated and further calcified by calcium salt precipitation

- X-ray Streak-or star-like scars with sharp edges and increased density

- Clinical Scar calcification stage

- To deterioration

○ Lesion extension

- There are exudation and necrosis around lesion

- X-ray unclear edge

- Clinical lesion with exudation

○ Dissolution and spread

- Liquefied necrosis discharged through natural tracts (bronchi,

---

- 小范围坏死吸收和消失

- **影像学** 增生边缘不清晰,密实,不均匀的云絮状阴影

- **临床** 需要治疗,采取措施

○ 纤维包裹和钙化

- **纤维包裹** 增生结核,渗出和小坏死灶机化,被纤维组织包囊

- **钙化** 大的坏死灶干燥、浓缩及钙盐沉淀进一步可发生钙化

- **X线** 条纹或星状,瘢痕,边缘清晰,密度增加

- **临床** 瘢痕钙化阶段

- 转向恶化

○ 浸润进展

- 病灶周围出现渗出和坏死

- **X线** 边界不清

- **临床** 病灶渗出

○ 溶解扩散

- 液化坏死通过自然管道(支气管,尿路等)排出腔道,形成

urinary tract and so on), forming cavity

- Lesion spreading by lymphatics, blood flow
- X-ray Density of shadow, inhomogeneous, bright region, and new focus
- Clinical Dissolution and spread stage

空腔

- 病变进入淋巴、血流分支播散

- X线 阴影不均匀，可见明亮区域，新旧病灶并存

- 临床 溶解和扩散阶段

Section 2 Pulmonary tuberculosis

第2节 肺结核

🔖 Primary pulmonary TB

Conception

- The first infection with tubercle bacillus in children and infants
- The infected persons have not had prior contact with the tubercle bacillus in teenage and adults

Pathological changes

- The characteristics of the lesion is primary complex under X-ray, showing dumbbell-like shadow
- Primary complex=Primary focus (Ghon focus) + Lymphangitis+ TB of hilar lymph nodes
- Primary focus Usually single, round, 1 ~ 1.5 cm area
  ○ Grossly Gray-yellow, consolidation

🔖 原发性肺结核

概述

- 儿童和婴儿第一次感染结核杆菌

- 青少年，成人尚未与结核杆菌接触的人的感染

病理特征

- 特征性表现是原发综合征，X线示哑铃状阴影

- 原发综合征=原发灶（Ghon灶）+淋巴管炎+肺门淋巴结结核

- 原发灶 单个，圆形，直径1～1.5厘米
  ○ 大体 灰黄色，坚固

- Location Lower part of the upper lobe or the upper part of the lower lobe, close to the pleura
- Lesion Caseous necrosis
- Lymphangitis
  - Uncommon
  - X-ray shows strip-like
  - Tubercle bacilli drained to lymphatics
- TB of hilar lymph nodes
  - Lymph nodes enlarged
  - X-ray Dumbbell shadow

Clinical features and Consequences
- Symptoms Slightly, no obvious signs
- Development and results
  - Natural healing Most patient (98%)
  - Small focus Absorption, fibrosis
  - Large focus Fibrous encapsulation and Calcification
- Deterioration and spread
  Cause
  - Children malnutrition or with influenza, measles
  - Adult with suppressed or defective immunity
- Routes of dissemination
  Spread By lymphatics
  - TB of hilar lymph nodes Tracheobronchial LN
  - Other LN mediastinal LN, post

- 部位 靠近胸膜的上叶下部或下叶上部
- 病变 干酪样坏死
- 淋巴管炎
  - 一般不可见
  - X线呈带状
  - 结核杆菌沿着淋巴管播散引起
- 肺门淋巴结核
  - 淋巴结肿大,干酪样坏死
  - X线 哑铃状阴影

临床特征与结局
- 体征 临床表现轻微,无明显症状
- 发展和结局
  - 自然愈合 大多数患者(98%)
  - 小病灶 吸收,纤维化
  - 大病灶 纤维包裹、钙化
- 恶化和传播
  原因
  - 儿童 营养不良或流行性感冒,麻疹
  - 成人 免疫力低下或虚弱
- 播散途径
  淋巴道转移
  - 肺门淋巴结结核,气管支气管淋巴结
  - 其他淋巴结 纵隔淋巴结,腹膜

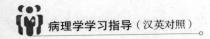

peritoneal LN, mesentery LN

Spread by bronchi

○ Children with bronchial hypoplasia are vulnerable to compression

○ Small bronchial diameter is easy to block

Spread by bloodstream

○ Tubercle bacilli enter bloodstream and lead to miliary TB of organs: lung, meninges, liver, spleen, kidney, adrenal glands

Secondary pulmonary TB

Conception

● Secondary pulmonary tuberculosis is referred to reinfections lesion of tubercle bacilli

● Usually involving adults, also called adult pulmonary TB

● Location　Initiated from apex of lung forming secondary focus

Pathogenesis

● Reinfection Causes

○ Endogenous reinfection primary pulmonary TB related

○ Exogenous reinfection not related to primary infection, TB spread by bloodstream

○ Extrapulmonary TB by blood to lung

● Pathological changes

○ Initial focus　Apex of the lung,

后淋巴结,肠系膜淋巴结

气管传播

○ 儿童支气管发育不全容易受压

○ 支气管直径小容易阻塞

血道传播

○ 结核杆菌进入血液流到达各器官造成血行扩散粟粒性结核,如肺、脑膜、肝、脾、肾、肾上腺等

继发性肺结核

概述

● 继发性肺结核是指再次感染结核杆菌导致的病变

● 通常为成年人,又叫成人型肺结核

● 位置　由肺尖开始形成继发性病灶

病理机制

● 再感染原因

○ 内源性再感染与原发性肺结核有关

○ 外源性再感染与原发感染无关,通过血液传播

○ 肺外结核通过血液到达肺

● 病理变化

○ 始发病灶　肺尖,局部抵抗力下

where is poorly ventilated and the immunity resistance decreased

○ Lesions

- When the patient has hypersensitivity and easily leading to caseous necrosis, liquefaction and cavity formation
- When the patient immune response is strong, the local lesions with hyperplasia leading to form tuberculosis nodules

○ Spread　Mainly through bronchi; Rarely spread through lymphatic fluid and bloodstream

- Clinical course

  ○ The lesion is lasting for a long time
  ○ They could become better or worse
  ○ The new and old lesions always coexist

Pathological types

- Focal pulmonary TB

  ○ It is early, inactive lesion
  ○ Apex 2～4 cm of right lung
  ○ Circumstance is clear
  ○ Diameter 0.5～1 cm
  ○ Pathological changes are proliferative tubercle and caseous necrosis
  ○ The results maybe fibrosis, calcification, or progress

- Infiltrative pulmonary TB

  ○ It is common type and active TB

降,通风不良

○ 病灶特点

- 机体过敏反应强时容易引起干酪样坏死,液化性坏死,形成空洞

- 机体免疫反应强时,病变局限伴增生形成结核结节

○ 播散　主要累及支气管;较少通过淋巴和血流播散

- 临床过程

  ○ 病变持续时间长
  ○ 好转或恶化
  ○ 新旧病灶混合存在

病理类型

- 局灶性肺结核

  ○ 早期无活性病变
  ○ 右肺尖下2～4厘米
  ○ 病灶边界清晰
  ○ 直径0.5～1厘米
  ○ 病理形态表现为增生性结核结节及干酪样坏死
  ○ 结局为纤维化、钙化或进展

- 浸润性肺结核

  ○ 是常见普通型活动性肺结核

○ Pathological changes showed exudative, caseous necrosis and inflammatory cells infiltration

○ Results mostly fibrosis or calcification

○ The cases with progression showed cavity formation, spread and develop to caseous pneumonia or chronic cavity

● Chronic fibro-cavitary pulmonary TB

○ Late stage, Open TB

○ Pathological changes Formation of thick wall:

Inner Caseous necrosis

Middle Tuberculous granulation

Outer Fibrous tissue

○ Features Bilateral lung, upper lobe of lung ,one or more, variation in size, irregular shape

○ Results Cirrhotic pulmonary TB

● Gaseous pneumonia

○ Disseminated by bronchi

○ Enlargement of lobe, Alveoli filled with serofibrinous exudates macrophages, caseous necrosis

○ Consolidation acute cavity

● Tuberculoma

○ Shape Solitary, fibrous encapsulated round, nodule with clear

○ 病变表现为渗出，干酪样坏死和炎细胞浸润

○ 结局 大部分纤维化或钙化

○ 进展病例形成空腔进展播散，发展为慢性纤维空洞TB或干酪性肺炎

● 慢性纤维空洞型肺结核

○ 慢纤洞是晚期开放性肺结核

○ 病理特征 厚壁空洞形成，空洞壁包括：

内 干酪样坏死

中 结核性肉芽肿

外 纤维组织

○ 特征 双侧肺肺上叶，一个或多个，大小不定，形状不规则，上旧下新

○ 结果 可能会发展为纤维性肺结核

● 干酪性肺炎

○ 由支气管传播

○ 肺叶弥漫性增大，肺泡腔充满渗出，巨噬细胞渗出和广泛的干酪样坏死

○ 合并急性空洞形成

● 结核瘤

○ 形状 孤立的，纤维包裹的圆形结节，边缘清晰，干酪样坏死灶

edge and caseous necrosis focus

- ○ Location   Upper lobe of the lung
- ○ Diameter   2～5 cm
- ○ Numbers   Usually one, sometime multiple

- ○ Easily misdiagnosed as tumor
- Tuberculous pleuritis
  - ○ Proliferative TB pleuritic   Foci below pleura extending directly, usually apex of lung, localized Proliferation adhesion
  - ○ Exsudative TB pleuritic Serofibrinous Inflammation, it can be absorbed completely, complication of pleural thicken and adhesion
- Miliary TB
  - ○ Acute miliary TB   It is common in child after primary pulmonary TB
  - ○ Chronic miliary TB   It is common in adult

Extrapulmonary TB

- Intestinal TB
  - ○ Intake through mouth, maybe milk
  - ○ Ulceration of Intestinal TB ulceration   Vertical to the long axis of intestine
  - ○ Primary complex   intestinal focus, mesentery lymph node TB
- Peritonitis of TB
- Meningitis of TB

- ○ 部位   肺上叶
- ○ 直径   2～5厘米
- ○ 数量   通常为一个, 有时多个

- ○ 易误诊为肿瘤
- 结核性胸膜炎
  - ○ 增生性结核性胸膜炎   结核病灶直接蔓延至胸膜下, 常出现在肺尖, 局部可以增生粘连

  - ○ 渗出性结核性胸膜炎   为纤维素性渗出性炎, 完全吸收, 可并发胸膜增厚和粘连

- 粟粒性结核
  - ○ 急性粟粒型肺结核   常见儿童, 继发于原发性肺结核
  - ○ 慢性粟粒型肺结核   成人常见

肺外结核

- 肠结核
  - ○ 消化道传播, 可能通过牛奶
  - ○ 肠结核溃疡与肠管长轴垂直, 容易引起肠狭窄

  - ○ 原发综合征   肠道病灶, 肠系膜淋巴结结核
- 结核性腹膜炎
- 结核性脑膜炎

- Genital and urology of TB
- Joint and bone of TB　Cold abscess
- Lymph node TB　Typical tubercle

- 生殖泌尿系统结核
- 骨关节结核　冷脓肿
- 淋巴结结核　典型结核结节

Section 3　Typhoid fever

第3节　伤寒

Conception

- Typhoid fever is acute proliferative inflammation involving mononuclear phagocytic system
- Clinical features
  - Fever
  - Bradycardia
  - Neutropenia
  - Spleen enlargement
  - Skin rose rash
- Spread
  - Source of infection　Patient and carrier
  - Fecal-oral route　Bacteria contaminating food or water infection by mouth

Pathogenesis

- Latent period 10 days
  - The bacteria phagocytized and reproduced in Lymph node of mesentery and spread into blood leads to bacteremia
- First week
  - Bacteria re-enter blood and releasing

概述

- 伤寒是累及全身单核巨噬细胞系统的急性增生性炎症

- 临床特征
  - 发热
  - 心动过缓
  - 中性粒细胞减少症
  - 脾大
  - 皮肤玫瑰皮疹
- 传播
  - 传染源　患者和携带者

  - 传播途径　粪–口途径,细菌污染食物或水而被感染

发病机制

- 潜伏期10天
  - 在肠系膜淋巴结,巨噬细胞吞噬并繁殖细菌进入血液引起菌血症

- 第1周
  - 细菌重新进入血液并释放内毒素

endotoxin to all over the body induce toxemia, septicemia (Vs pyemia) leading typhoid symptoms and lesions

- 2～3 week
  - Typhoid bacilli reproducing in gallbladder enter LN of intestinal tract and leads severe sensitive reaction with intestinal necrosis and ulceration
- Fourth weeks
  - Immunity　Healing gradually
  - LN of intestine (ileum)　LN of mesentery, liver, spleen and bone marrow are gradually recovery

Pathological Features

- Formation of typhoid granuloma
  - Typhoid cell　Macrophage which phagocytized RBC, bacilli, lymphocyte and cell debris
  - Typhoid granuloma　Typhoid cells aggregated to form small nodule
  - Infiltrate cells　Many of lymphocyte and rarely neutrophils

Intestinal tract lesions

- Location　Terminal ileum is the most commonly affected location of intestinal typhoid
- Stages　The lesion can be divided to 4 stages

到达全身引起毒血症, 败血病 (脓毒败血症), 引起伤寒的相应症状和病变

- 第2～3周
  - 伤寒杆菌在胆囊中繁殖, 排出, 再次到达肠壁淋巴结引起严重致敏反应, 导致肠黏膜坏死, 溃疡

- 第4周
  - 免疫力　逐渐恢复
  - 肠 (回肠)　肠系膜淋巴结、肝、脾、骨髓等逐渐恢复

病理特征

- 伤寒肉芽肿的形成
  - 伤寒细胞　吞噬了RBC, 伤寒杆菌, 淋巴细胞和细胞碎片的巨噬细胞
  - 伤寒肉芽肿　伤寒细胞聚集形成的小结节
  - 浸润细胞　以淋巴细胞为主, 中性粒细胞较少

肠道病变

- 位置　肠道病变主要位于回肠末端

- 分期　可分4期

Stage 1   Gyrus like swelling stage
              Hyperplasia of Peyer's patch
  ○ The first week of the onset
  ○ Features   Proliferation of macrophage and formation of typhoid granuloma
  ○ Grossly   There are oval patches which run along the axes of the intestine, show as button like protrusion
  ○ Location   The lymphoid tissue of intestinal tract, Peyer's nodules of ileum and solitary lymph follicles of cecum

Stage 2   Necrotic stage
  ○ The second week of the onset
  ○ Hypersensitive reaction to toxins, macrophages proliferate and compress capillaries, leading to vascular thrombosis, ischemia and necrosis
  ○ Grossly   The lesion shows necrosis at center with swelling margin

Stage 3   Ulcerative stage
  ○ The third week of the onset
  ○ Cause   Necrosis
  ○ Grossly   Ileal nodules (Peyer's nodes) ulcers are oval in shape, the long axis of the ulcer is parallel to the long axis of the bowel, solitary

第 1 期　髓样肿胀期
          集合淋巴小结增生
  ○ 发病的第 1 周
  ○ 特征　巨噬细胞增生形成伤寒肉芽肿

  ○ 大体　沿肠管长轴延伸的椭圆形斑块，看似纽扣样凸起

  ○ 位置　空肠孤立淋巴小结和回肠集合淋巴小结

第 2 期　坏死期
  ○ 发病的第 2 周
  ○ 对内毒素敏感反应，巨噬细胞增生压迫毛细血管导致血管血栓形成，缺血并坏死

  ○ 大体　病变中央坏死，边缘肿胀

第 3 期　溃疡期
  ○ 发病的第 3 周
  ○ 原因　坏死
  ○ 大体　回肠集合淋巴小结溃疡呈椭圆形，溃疡的长轴与肠管长轴平行，孤立淋巴小结溃疡是小的圆形溃疡

lymph node ulcers are small round

- ○ Complication   Hemorrhage and perforation

Stage 4   Healing stage

- ○ The fourth week of the onset
- ○ Granulation tissue repair by scar
- ○ No intestinal tract obstruction because of ulcer is parallel with the long axis of intestinal tract

Lesions in other organs

- Lesion in other mononuclear phagocyte system
  - ○ Lymph node of mesentery Typhoid granuloma and little necrosis
  - ○ Spleen   Moderate enlargement, macrophage proliferation forming granuloma, necrosis
  - ○ Liver   Enlargement and become soft, granuloma, necrosis, monocyte or lymphocyte infiltration
  - ○ Bone marrow   Macrophage proliferation, granuloma and necrosis. The numbers of neutrophil and eosinophil are decreased
- Gall bladder
  - ○ The typhoid bacilli reproduce easily in gallbladder with mild inflammation and lesion
  - ○ The bacteria can exist in gallbladder after healing for a long time as

---

- ○ 并发症   可伴出血和穿孔

第4期   恢复期

- ○ 疾病的第4周
- ○ 肉芽组织修复形成瘢痕
- ○ 溃疡修复后无肠狭窄,原因是溃疡与肠管长轴平行

其他器官中的病变

- 其他单核吞噬细胞系统
  - ○ 肠系膜淋巴结   伤寒肉芽肿和小灶坏死
  - ○ 脾脏   中度肿大,巨噬细胞增生形成肉芽肿,坏死
  - ○ 肝脏   肿大,质地柔软,肉芽肿形成,坏死,单核细胞或淋巴细胞浸润
  - ○ 骨髓   巨噬细胞增生和肉芽肿形成,坏死,中性粒细胞和嗜酸性细胞下降
- 胆囊
  - ○ 伤寒杆菌容易在胆囊中繁殖,仅出现轻度炎症和病变
  - ○ 胆囊病变治愈后,细菌仍然会存在很长时间,称为慢性病菌携带

chronic carrier (Typhoid Mary)

- Myocardium
  - There are cloudy swelling and necrosis
  - Bradycardia　because of toxic myocarditis leads to bradycardia
- Kidney
  - Epithelial cell of fallopian tube are swelling
  - Immune complex nephritis
- Skin
  - Rose spots Reticuloendothelial involvement of the chest, back, and abdomen forms rosettes
- Muscles
  - There was coagulative necrosis in diaphragm muscle, rectus abdominis and adductor thigh showed coagulative necrosis looks like wax degeneration

Clinical results

- Mainly healing, there are little complication
- Complications
  - Hemorrhage　shock
  - Perforation　Diffuse peritonitis
  - Lobular pneumonia　There are secondary diseases when resistance of human body is decreased, such as lobular pneumonia
  - Infection of the other organs　Bone

者（伤寒玛丽）

- 心肌
  - 心肌呈云絮样肿胀和坏死
  - **心动过缓**　中毒性心肌炎导致心动过缓
- 肾脏
  - 输尿管上皮浑浊肿胀
  - 免疫复合物性肾炎
- 皮肤
  - 胸部、背部、腹部网状内皮受累形成玫瑰斑
- 肌肉
  - 膈肌，腹直肌，大腿内收肌呈凝固性坏死（蜡样变性）

临床结局

- 大部分能治愈，无并发症

- 并发症
  - **出血**　导致休克
  - **穿孔**　引起弥漫性腹膜炎
  - **小叶性肺炎**　当机体抵抗力下降时可以引起其他继发性疾病如小叶性肺炎
  - **其他器官感染**　如骨髓，关节，脑

marrow, joint, meninges, and kidney

- **Death** Septicemia, hemorrhage, perforation

膜和肾脏

- **死亡** 败血症,出血,穿孔

Section 4 Bacillary dysentery

第4节 细菌性痢疾

Conception

- Bacillary dysentery is an infectious disease of intestinal tract caused by dysentery bacilli (Gram negative bacillus)
- Usually endemic in summer and autumn
- It belongs to fibrinous inflammation
- Incidence of the disease children > adult (20～39 years) > old people

概述

- 由痢疾杆菌引起的消化道传染病(G-)

- 多发于夏、秋季
- 属于急性纤维性炎
- **发病率** 儿童＞20～39岁成人＞老年

Etiology and pathogenesis

- Pathogen
  - Dysentery bacilli (Gram negative) are short rod bacteria and secret endotoxin
  - Virulence flexneri > sonnei > boydii > shigella
- Source of infection
  - Patient
  - Carrier
- Routes of infection
  - The contaminated food, water, kitchen utensils, hand of bacillus,

病因和病机

- **病原体**
  - 痢疾杆菌(革兰阴性),短杆菌通过内毒素致病

  - **毒力** 福氏＞宋内氏＞鲍氏＞志贺菌
- **感染源**
  - 患者
  - 带菌者
- **感染途径**
  - 被污染的食物、水、厨房用具和手经口食入

enter the body through mouth

- Pathogenesis
  - Bacilli were killed by gastric acid in stomach or rejected by normal bacteria group in intestinal tract
  - Some patient has occult infection without sign because of SIgA
  - When human body exhausted or resistance decreased due to chronic disease, there will be bacillary dysentery onset
  - The mainly pathogenic factor is bacilli with strong invading ability and endotoxins

Type of Lesion

Acute bacillary dysentery

- Location   Large intestine, especially left colon, rectum
- Early stage   Acute catarrh inflammation showed mucosa congestion, edema, neutrophil and macrophage
- Progression   Pseudomembranous inflammation
- Pseudo-membrane   Made of fibrin, necrotic tissue, neutrophils, RBC and bacilli
- Ulcer feature   The gyrus-like material at the top of the intestinal mucosal fold falls off, fuses into a fragmented pseudo-membrane. The fall-off area forms a

- 发病机制
  - 机体抵抗力正常时，痢疾杆菌被食入胃会被胃酸杀死，到达肠道也会被正常菌群排斥
  - 部分人为隐匿性感染由于SIgA功能降低
  - 机体患有慢性病，疲劳过度，抵抗力下降易患病

  - 主要致病因子是细菌的侵袭能力和内毒素

病变类型

急性细菌性痢疾

- 部位   主要累及大肠，尤其是左半结肠、直肠
- 早期   急性卡他炎，表现为黏液分泌，黏膜充血水肿，中性粒细胞和巨噬细胞浸润
- 进展   伪膜性炎
- 假膜   由纤维蛋白、坏死组织、中性粒细胞、红细胞和痢疾杆菌构成
- 溃疡特点   肠黏膜皱襞顶部脑回样物质脱落、融合成碎片状假膜，脱落形成地图状浅表溃疡

superficial map-like ulcer

- Signs and Symptoms
  - Fever, Headache, Fatigue, Abdominal pain, Diarrhea, Pus-mucin-blood mixed stools, Tenesmus
- Results
  - Healing   Mostly recovery in 1～2 weeks
  - Complications   There is no perforation and hemorrhage

Chronic bacillary dysentery

Conception

- Clinical course of disease lasts more than two months
- Mostly are from acute bacillary dysentery

Clinical features

- Abdominal pain, Diarrhea, Mucus stool, abdominal distension

Clinical results

- The course of the disease persisted for a long time
- Chronic carrier is a source of infection

Toxic bacillary dysentery

Conception

- Acute onset
- Toxic symptoms are very prominent and severe
- Symptoms of intestinal canal is slight
- Usually 2～7 years of age

- 体征和症状
  - 发热，头痛，疲劳，腹痛，腹泻，黏液脓血便，里急后重

- 结局
  - 治愈   病程最长 1～2 周
  - 并发症   一般无穿孔和出血

慢性细菌性痢疾

概述

- 临床病程＞2个月
- 多数是由于急性细菌性痢疾

临床特征

- 腹痛，腹泻，黏液便，腹胀

临床结局

- 病程长期持续
- 慢性病菌携带者成为感染源

中毒性细菌性痢疾

概述

- 急性发作
- 中毒症状非常突出和严重
- 肠道症状轻微
- 通常发生在 2～7 岁

Bacteria

- Flexner and Sonnei group of bacteria

Pathological changes

- Inflammatory change in the colon is rather slight catarrh with mucus secretion
- Sometimes shows follicular enteritis

Clinical features

- The symptoms are severe, there are fever, DIC and shock
- But the signs of digestive tract are slightly

Clinical Results

- The course of the disease is different
- Serious   DIC and shock

病原菌

- 福氏菌和宋内氏菌

病理变化

- 结肠炎轻微，黏膜炎症较轻，仅仅黏液分泌增多

- 有时类似滤泡性肠炎

临床特征

- 全身中毒症状很重，发热，弥散性血管内凝血甚至休克
- 消化道的症状轻微

临床结局

- 病程不同
- **严重者**　弥散性血管内凝血和休克

Section 5   Parasitosis

Amoebiasis

Conception

- Amoebiasis is an infectious diseases caused by the Entameba hislytica
- Infection occurs by ingestion of cysts of Entameba hislytica in food and water contaminated with feces
- The protozoan of Entameba hislytica may penetrate the mucosa and invade local tissue or spread to other organs: liver, lung, brain or skin

第5节   寄生虫病

阿米巴病

概述

- 阿米巴病是由溶组织阿米巴虫引起的传染性疾病
- 人因食入被粪便污染的食物和水中的阿米巴包囊而导致感染

- 溶组织阿米巴寄生在肠道中，穿透肠黏膜，侵入局部组织或扩散到其他器官如肝、肺、脑或皮肤

Intestinal Amoebiasis

Etiology and Pathogenesis

- E. histolytica is well recognized as a pathogenic ameba, associated with intestinal and extraintestinal infections
- E. histolytica is transmitted when humans swallow mature cysts in food, water, or hands contaminated by feces
- After cyst ingestion by humans, there is no changes in an acid environment of stomach. The cyst is destroyed by the alkaline intestinal medium after entering into intestinal tract
- The encysted organism becomes to four separated small trophozoites and develop into adult large trophozoites
- Ameba have enzymes which can lyse host tissue and forming ulceration in intestinal tract

Pathological changes

- Multiple areas of enzymatic necrosis of tissue and acute inflammation leading to mucosal ulcer throughout the colon
- Most lesions are located in right colon, especially ileocecal junction
- Ulcers are raised as "flask-shaped", mucosal surface between ulcer looks like healthy mucosa
- Microscopically An ulcer reveals

肠阿米巴病

病因和发病机制

- 溶组织性阿米巴被公认是一种致病性阿米巴原虫,与肠道和肠外感染均有关
- 粪便污染了食物,水或手,人们通过食入其中的成熟包囊而传播疾病
- 人误食溶组织性阿米巴包囊后,在胃的酸性环境中未发生变化,到达肠道碱性环境,包囊则破坏
- 包囊内的生物体变成了四个阿米巴小滋养体,并发展成为成熟的大滋养体
- 阿米巴含破坏宿主组织的酶,导致肠道溃疡形成

病理变化

- 整个结肠黏膜溃疡形成,由阿米巴分泌的溶解酶引起组织坏死和急性炎症
- 大部分病变位于右半结肠,尤其是回盲部
- 溃疡看上去较小,呈纽扣样,呈"烧瓶状"状,溃疡之间的黏膜表面看起来像健康的肠黏膜
- 镜下 可见由寄生虫的蛋白水解酶

necrosis caused by parasites' proteolytic enzymes. Amebas are found in the walls of the ulcers

引起的坏死和出血，溃疡壁上可见阿米巴滋养体

- Inflammation usually does not occur unless there has been secondary bacterial infection

- 除非发生继发性细菌感染，否则通常不会发生急性炎症

Clinical features

临床特征

- Intestinal amebiasis is often called amebic dysentery

- 肠阿米巴病通常称为阿米巴痢疾

- The patients present with bloody and mucous diarrhea with jam-like stool

- 出现黏液血性腹泻，果酱样便

- The patient always has low fever

- 患者常有低热

Extra-intestinal Amoebiasis

肠外阿米巴病

Amoebic liver abscess

阿米巴肝脓肿

Conception

概述

- Hepatic amebiasis is the most common complication of intestinal infection by E. histolytica

- 肝阿米巴病是溶组织性阿米巴感染肠道最常见的并发症

- It is caused by the entry of amebic trophozoites into portal venous radicles in the colonic submucosa

- 由阿米巴滋养体进入结肠黏膜下门静脉小分支进入肝脏而引起

- It shows as amoebic liver abscess

- 常表现为阿米巴肝脓肿

Pathological changes

病理变化

- Grossly

- 大体

  ○ Amebic abscesses are large, lined by an irregular wall containing amebic "pus"

  ○ 阿米巴肝脓肿较大，脓肿壁不规则，含有阿米巴"脓液"

  ○ Abscesses compress adjacent liver tissue

  ○ 脓肿压迫周围肝组织

  ○ Pseudocapsule is around abscess with invasive margin

  ○ 脓肿周围可见假包膜，边缘呈浸润性

- Microscopically
  - Abscess is made of lots of pus with necrosis
  - Amebic trophozoites are found in the walls of the abscess
  - There are no inflammation cells in the walls of the abscess

Clinical features

- Right upper quadrant pain, hepatomegaly
- Low fever
- Weight loss
- Night sweats

Other organ amoebida

- Amebic lung abscess
  - Direct extension from hepatic abscesses
- Amebic brain abscess
  - Usually solitary and located either cerebral hemisphere which is spread by blood

Schistosomiasis

Conception

- Schistosomiasis is caused by Schistosoma Japonicum in China
- Schistosomiasis is mainly distributed in drainage area of Yangtze River
- Schistosomiasis was controlled after establishment of new China

Etiology and Pathogenesis

- The infection is transmitted by

- 镜下
  - 脓肿内含大量脓性坏死组织
  - 脓肿壁可见阿米巴滋养体
  - 脓肿内没有炎细胞

临床特征

- 右上腹疼痛,肝大
- 低热
- 体重减轻
- 盗汗

其他器官的阿米巴

- 阿米巴肺脓肿
  - 肝脓肿直接蔓延所致
- 阿米巴脑脓肿
  - 通常为孤立性,位于大脑半球,为血道播散

血吸虫病

概述

- 中国血吸虫病是由日本血吸虫感染引起
- 血吸虫病主要分布在我国长江流域
- 新中国成立后血吸虫病得到有效控制

病因和病机

- 人类感染血吸虫是血吸虫尾蚴钻入

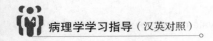

penetration of cercariae of Schistosoma Japonicum through human intact skin

人完整的皮肤而传播

- Once the cercariae have successfully entered the host, it is termed a schistosomulum

- 一旦尾蚴成功地进入宿主体内就称为血吸虫童虫

- The schistosomulum migrates through the tissues and finally invades a blood vessel leading Schistosomiasis

- 血吸虫童虫通过组织迁移最终侵入血管引起血吸虫病

Pathological feature

病理学特征

- Lesions caused by cercariae
  ○ It is signalled by petechial haemorrhages and edema

- 尾蚴引起的病变
  ○ 皮肤出现出血点，伴有水肿

  ○ Lasting for two to five days
  ○ Then disappear naturally

  ○ 持续2～5天
  ○ 然后自然消失

- Lesions caused by schistosomulum
  ○ The schistosomulum expresses antigens on its surface leads host immune response providing some degree of resistance to reinfection

- 童虫引起的病变
  ○ 血吸虫童虫表面会表达抗原导致宿主免疫反应，对再感染具有一定程度的抵抗力

- Lesions caused by adult worms
  ○ The adult worms do not cause severe damage and immune response to the host

- 成虫引起的病变
  ○ 成虫不会对宿主造成严重损害和免疫反应

- Lesions caused by eggs   The main lesion of Schistosomiasis is caused by eggs

- 虫卵引起的病变   血吸虫病的主要病变由虫卵所致

  ○ Acute egg nodule
  Also called eosinophilic Granuloma The eggs are trapped in the tissue leading severe allergic reaction, cellular infiltrates include lots

  ○ 急性虫卵结节
  又称嗜酸性肉芽肿，由血吸虫虫卵沉积到组织中引起的反应，虫卵中的毛蚴引起过敏反应形成肉芽肿，可见较多嗜酸性粒细胞浸

of eosinophils, lymphocytes, macrophages, and fibroblast

○ Chronic egg nodule

Also known as pseudo-tubercular nodules. It is a typical chronic granuloma. Chronic egg nodules result from the deposition of old schistosome eggs, causing foreign body giant cell hyperplasia, lymphocytic infiltration, and fibrous tissue hyperplasia

Colonic Schistosomiasis

- Location Involving distal parts of the colon, left colon and rectum
- Grossly Intestine wall becomes inflamed and thickened, there are many polyps in intestinal tract. During heavy infection, the colon wall becomes rigid leading to mechanical obstruction
- Microscopically There are acute egg nodule and chronic egg nodule

Hepatosplenic Schistosomiasis

- The eggs of schistosomiasis deposited in the portal triads of the liver stimulate a granulomatous response, leading to continuous fibrosis of the periportal tissue
- Schistosoma cirrhosis Portal system is totally replaced by granuloma and fibrosis, called "pipestem" fibrosis

润,以及淋巴细胞、巨噬细胞和成纤维细胞浸润

○ **慢性虫卵结节**

又称假结核结节,是典型的慢性肉芽肿。慢性虫卵结节由陈旧性血吸虫卵沉积引起异物巨细胞增生、淋巴细胞浸润和纤维组织增生

结肠血吸虫病

- **部位** 结肠远端,左半结肠,尤其乙状结肠和直肠
- **大体** 肠壁增厚,可见息肉形成,严重者肠壁僵硬或梗阻

- **镜下** 可见急性虫卵结节和慢性虫卵结节

肝血吸虫病

- 血吸虫卵沉积在肝门管区刺激机体产生肉芽肿反应,导致门静脉周围组织持续纤维化

- **血吸虫肝硬化** 肝门管系统完全被肉芽肿和纤维化所取代,又称干线性肝硬化

- Periportal fibrosis and vascular destruction leads to portal hypertension, splenomegaly, ascites and the development of collateral circulation

- 周围肝纤维化和血管走形异常导致门脉高压,脾肿大和侧支循环的形成

Section 6　Central nervous system disease

第6节　中枢神经系统疾病

Epidemic cerebrospinal meningitis

流行性脑脊髓膜炎

Etiology and pathogenesis

- Pathogenic organisms
  - Teenagers and youth, meningococcal
  - Infant, bacillus coli
  - < 3 years, influenza bacilli
  - Senile, pneumococcus
- Route of infection
  - Respiratory tract by droplets
  - When human resistance is normal: Local inflammation as a carrier
  - When human resistance is decreased: the bacteria enter blood and reproduce, leading to meningitis
  - Bloodstream spread accounts for the majority of cases by respiratory tract, skin or intestine

Pathological changes

- Acute purulent inflammation (surface purulence)
- Involving brain convex surface around

病因与发病机制

- 病原体
  - 青少年,青年,脑膜炎球菌
  - 婴儿,大肠杆菌
  - < 3 岁小儿,流感杆菌
  - 老年人,肺炎球菌
- 传播途径
  - 呼吸道飞沫
  - 机体抵抗力正常时仅形成局部炎症,成为携带者
  - 机体抵抗力低时细菌入血并繁殖,引起脑膜炎

  - 呼吸道、皮肤及消化道感染者大部分通过血道传播

病理变化

- 急性化脓性炎症（表面化脓）

- 累及额叶和顶叶脑皮质表面及大脑

sagittal sinus of frontal and parietal lobe

- Grossly
  - Meninge is highly congested
  - Subarachnoid space is filled up with purulent exudate
- Microscopically
  - Subarachnoid space is filled with exudations of neutrophils, fibrin, monocyte and lymphocyte
  - The blood vessel is congested and cerebral convex has mild edema

Results and complications

- Most patients will be recovered if treatment is placed in time
- Hydrocephalus　Due to the blockage of circulation of cerebrospinal fluid by adhered meninges
- There is no nervous damage. Ischemia and infarct of brain are rare

Burst meningitis

- A type of burst meningitis suddenly onset in children with burst meningococcal septicemia
- Also called Warterhouse-Friederichsen Syndrome
- Mechanism of the lesion is endotoxin by bacteria and DIC
- The patient has hemorrhage of both sides of brain, failure of adrenocortical

基底部

- 大体
  - 脑膜高度淤血
  - 蛛网膜下腔充满脓性渗出液

- 镜下
  - 蛛网膜下腔充满中性粒细胞、纤维蛋白、单核细胞和淋巴细胞

  - 血管淤血，而脑组织轻度水肿

结局和并发症

- 如及时治疗大部分患者能恢复

- 脑积水　脑膜粘连阻塞脑脊液循环

- 无神经系统损伤，很少出现缺血和脑梗死

暴发性脑膜炎

- 一种儿童型脑膜炎，突然发生脑膜炎双球菌性败血症

- 又称为沃-佛综合征

- 发病机制是细菌释放内毒素导致弥散性血管内凝血
- 出现双侧肾上腺出血，肾上腺皮质功能衰竭，循环障碍，皮肤紫癜和休克

function and circulation, skin purpura and shock

Clinical Features

- Acute meningitis presents with fever
- Symptoms of meningeal irritation, which include headache, neck pain, and vomiting
- Physical examination reveals neck stiffness and a positive Kernig's sign
- In general, bacterial meningitis is a serious disease with considerable risk of death

Prognosis

- Most patients have good prognosis
- More than 90% patients can be healing
- The complications are rare
- Severe meningitis with poor prognosis

Epidemic encephalitis B

Etiology and pathogenesis

- **Pathogen** Encephalitis virus B from Japanese, it is RNA virus
- **Transmitted Routes** Vertical transmission, Animal-mosquito-animal
- **Mediator vectors** Mosquitoes
- **Intermediate hosts** Horses, cattle, pigs
- Mosquitoes bite an infected middle host and spread the virus by biting human person

临床特征

- 急性脑膜炎伴发热
- 脑膜刺激征，包括头痛、颈部疼痛和呕吐

- 体格检查显示颈项强直和克氏征阳性
- 细菌性脑膜炎是一种严重的急性传染病，有相当大的死亡风险

预后

- 多数病人预后良好
- 90%以上患者能痊愈

- 并发症相对较少
- 严重脑膜炎预后差

流行性乙型脑炎

病因病机

- **病原体** 日本的乙型脑炎病毒，属于RNA病毒
- **传播途径** 动物—蚊子—人（垂直传播）
- **传播媒介** 蚊子
- **中间宿主** 马、牛、猪

- 蚊子叮咬了感染病毒的中间宿主，又叮咬人而传播

- Whether the virus causes the disease depends on the functional status of human cellular immune response and blood-brain barrier

Pathological changes

- Epidemic encephalitis B is an alterative inflammation involving cerebral convex
- Location   Cerebral cortex and basal ganglia
- Grossly   Meninges congestion, edema, millet cerebral dialysis focus
- Microscopically

  Inflammatory reaction

  ○ Disorder of local circulation, highly congestion of blood vessels
  ○ Perivascular cuffing   Lymphocyte, monocyte infiltrating around vessels

  Injury of neuron

  ○ Degeneration Cell Neuron swelling and Nissl body disappear
  ○ Necrosis   Red neuron, ghost cell
  ○ Soften foci   Necrotic foci, soften foci, lacunar infarct

  Injury of neuroglia

  ○ Proliferation of astrocyte, oligodendrocyte, microglia
  ○ Neuronophagia   Necrotic neuron cell was phagocytized by microglia or macrophage

- 病毒是否引起疾病取决于人体细胞免疫反应和血脑屏障的功能状态

病理变化

- 流行性乙型脑炎是累及脑实质的变质性炎症

- 部位   中枢神经系统脑实质,大脑皮质和基底节
- 大体   脑膜充血、水肿,可见粟粒样软化灶
- 镜下

  炎症反应

  ○ 局部血液循环障碍,血管高度充血
  ○ 血管袖套   血管周围淋巴细胞、单核细胞浸润

  神经元损伤

  ○ 细胞变性   神经元肿胀,尼氏小体消失
  ○ 坏死   红色神经元,鬼影细胞
  ○ 软化灶   脑坏死,软化病灶,腔隙性脑梗死

  神经胶质细胞损伤

  ○ 星形胶质细胞,少突胶质细胞,室管膜细胞,小胶质细胞等增生
  ○ 噬神经细胞现象   坏死神经元被小胶质细胞或巨噬细胞吞噬的现象

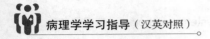

- Satellitosis   A neuron cell surrounded by more than 5 oligodendrocytes
- Microglial nodule   Microglia cell proliferative nodule
- Gitter cell   Foam cell

Clinical and Prognosis

- Endemic season   Summer and autumn, more in July to September
- Clinical features   High fever and coma
- Complicates   Most patient have dysfunction of brain
- The prognosis is poor

Section 7   Sexually transmitted disease (STD)

Conception

- Transmitted by sex intersection related contact action
- Most have human papillomavirus infection

Gonorrhea

Conception

- Gonorrhea is a purulent inflammation of mucosa surfaces caused by a sexually transmitted
- It can cause urethritis, cervicitis, epididymitis, pharyngitis, proctitis,

---

- 卫星灶   一个神经细胞周围有5个以上的少突胶质细胞围绕
- 小胶质细胞结节   小胶质细胞增生形成结节状
- 格子细胞   泡沫细胞

临床与预后

- 季节性   多发生于夏、秋季,7～9月多见
- 临床特征   高热和昏迷
- 并发症   大多数患者有脑功能障碍
- 预后差

第7节   性传播疾病

概述

- 性传播疾病主要通过性交或其相关的接触传播
- 多数有人乳头瘤病毒感染

淋病

概述

- 淋病是性传播引起的黏膜表面化脓性炎症
- 引起尿道炎,宫颈炎,附睾炎,咽炎,直肠炎和盆腔炎

and pelvic inflammation

Etiology

- Pathogen   Neisseria gonorrhoeae;
- The bacteria is easily infecting urinary and genital epithelial cells

Pathological changes

- Grossly   Purulent secretion
- Microscopically   Neutrophil infiltration and necrotic neutrophil forming pus

Prognosis

- Most gonococcal infections respond quickly to antibiotic therapy

Condyloma acuminata

Conception

- Also called venereal or genital warts
- It is associated with papillomavirus (HPV), especially type 6 and 11
- Location   Perianal region, vulva, penis, vagina, cervix, larynx, skin and mouth
- Latent time   About 3 months

Pathological changes

- Grossly
  - Typical condyloma usually shows a discrete papillary growth pattern that arises from a single stalk as cauliflower shape
- Microscopically
  - Squamous papilloma-like hyperplasia characterized by marked hyperkeratosis, acanthosis and

病因

- 病原体   淋球菌
- 淋球菌容易感染泌尿生殖道上皮

病理特征

- 大体   脓性分泌物
- 镜下   中性粒细胞浸润,中性粒细胞坏死形成脓液

预后

- 大多数淋球菌感染对抗生素治疗反应好

尖锐湿疣

概述

- 也称为生殖器疣
- 与人类乳头状瘤病毒(HPV)相关,尤其是6型和11型
- 部位   肛周、外阴、阴茎、阴道、子宫颈、喉、皮肤、口等
- 潜伏时间   约3个月

病理特征

- 大体
  - 典型的尖锐湿疣通常是单个蒂的乳头状生长方式,似菜花样
- 镜下
  - 鳞状上皮呈乳头状瘤样增生伴有明显角化过度,棘细胞层增生明显

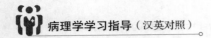

hyperplasia of the prickle cell layer

○ Koilocytosis is commonly observed in the superficial epithelial cells with perinuclear cytoplasmic halos

○ A chronic inflammatory infiltrate is often observed within the dermis

○ The growth papillary is usually characteristically upward toward the surface and not downward into the tissue

Prognosis

● The patients always don't have signs

● During pregnancy, the illness often becomes active and worse

● Many patients fail to respond to treatment, or recurrent after adequate response to condyloma acuminate

Syphilis

Etiology

● Pathogen　The spirochaete treponema pallidum

● It is a delicate corkscrew-shaped bacillus

● Syphilis was first infected from Europe and is said to be related to the discovery of new continent by Christopher Columbus

Pathogenesis

● Syphilis can be classified as acquired syphilis and congenital syphilis

● It is transmitted in 3 ways of acquired

○ 乳头表层细胞可见挖空细胞，核周可见胞浆空晕

○ 真皮内可见慢性炎细胞浸润，以淋巴细胞为主

○ 乳头通常朝着表面向上生长而不是向下进入组织

预后

● 经常无症状

● 在怀孕期间生长活跃且恶化

● 许多患者对治疗无反应，或对尖锐湿疣治疗反应后仍复发

梅毒

病因

● 病原体　梅毒螺旋体

● 是一种精致的螺旋形杆菌

● 梅毒首先从欧洲开始，据说与哥伦布发现新大陆有关

发病机制

● 梅毒可分为获得性梅毒和先天性梅毒

● 在获得性梅毒中，它以3种方式传播

syphilis

- ○ The most common way is from intimate sexually contacting with infectious lesions
- ○ The second is from blood transfusions
- ○ The third is transplacental from an infected mother to her fetus

Basic pathological changes

- Small blood vessel disease
  - ○ Obliterating endarteritis
  - ○ Periarteritis lymphocyte and plasma cell infiltration
- Granuloma
  - ○ Gumma It is large mass that may be mistaken for a neoplasm
  - ○ It is an area of rubbery coagulative necrosis in the central area surrounded by epithelioid cells, lymphocytes, numerous plasma cells, and fibrosis

Clinical Stage

- The incubation time of syphilis is about 21～28 days
- The antibody to syphilis was produced after infected 6 week
- There are three stage of syphilis: primary, secondary and tertiary syphilis
- The early syphilis consist of primary and secondary syphilis, and tertiary syphilis is late syphilis

- ○ 最常见的方式是通过与梅毒患者亲密的性接触
- ○ 第二是通过输血感染
- ○ 第三是从受感染的母亲通过胎盘传给胎儿

基本病理变化

- 小血管疾病
  - ○ 闭塞性动脉内膜炎
  - ○ 小动脉周围炎 小动脉周围淋巴细胞、浆细胞浸润
- 肉芽肿
  - ○ 梅毒树胶肿 是一种较大的肿块,容易误诊为肿瘤
  - ○ 肿块中央是橡胶状凝固性坏死,周围有上皮样细胞、淋巴细胞、大量浆细胞和纤维化组织

临床分期

- 梅毒潜伏期为21～28天
- 机体感染6周后产生梅毒抗体
- 梅毒分三期:一期、二期和三期梅毒
- 早期梅毒包括一期和二期梅毒,三期梅毒属于晚期梅毒

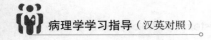

- Stage 1　Primary syphilis, more contagious
  - Develop after 3 weeks by infected
  - Chancre or Hard chancre　Painless solitary papule or nodule, with inflammation perivascular mainly infiltrating by plasma cell and lymphocyte
- Stage 2　Secondary syphilis, more contagious
  - Develop after 7 to 8 weeks by infected
  - May begin with primary chancre healed
  - Patient have fever, malaise and lymph node enlarged
  - Rose rash　face or palm with red colour
  - Lymph node enlargement Lymphatic spread follows predictable routes according to the site of the lesion; inguinal lymph nodes are the primary affected
  - The symptoms and the lesions are easily disappeared spontaneously over a few months
- Stage 3　Tertiary syphilis, less contagious
  - Develop after 4 to 5 years or more by infected
  - Typical lesion is gumma

- 一期梅毒　传染性强
  - 感染后3周发生
  - 下疳或硬下疳　无痛性单个丘疹或结节，主要为血管周围大量浆细胞及淋巴细胞炎

- 二期梅毒　传染性强
  - 发生在感染后7~8周
  - 可能在一期下疳愈合时就已经开始
  - 病人常有发热、萎靡和淋巴结肿大
  - 玫瑰疹　多位于脸部和手掌，颜色较红
  - 淋巴结肿大　与病变部位淋巴引流有关，腹股沟淋巴结最常受影响
  - 病变和体征容易在几个月内自发消退

- 三期梅毒　传染性小
  - 发生在梅毒感染后4~5年或更久
  - 典型病变为梅毒树胶肿

○ It is always involving the aorta and central nervous system, causing fibrosis and organ deformation

Acquired immunodeficiency syndrome (AIDS)

- AIDS is a syndrome that represents the most severe form of infection with the retrovirus HIV
- Epidemiology of AIDS has clearly delineated the mechanisms of spread as sexual intercourse, transfer of blood, and vertical transfer from infected mother to newborn child
- There is no available means of reversing the immune deficiency because of destroyed of CD4 positive T lymphocytes
- Opportunistic infections, uncommon malignant neoplasms, and intractable immune deficiency are hallmarks and severe secondary complications of AIDS
- Therapy is restricted to treating the complicating infections and tumors

○ 常累及主动脉和中枢神经系统，引起纤维化和器官变形

获得性免疫缺陷综合征（艾滋病）

- 艾滋病是一种逆转录艾滋病病毒感染引起的免疫缺陷综合征

- 艾滋病流行病学显示艾滋病的传播机制，包括性交、血液传播和母婴垂直传播

- 艾滋病致病机制是由于CD4$^+$T淋巴细胞的破坏而导致无法逆转的免疫缺陷

- 机会性感染、罕见恶性肿瘤和难治性免疫缺陷是艾滋病的特征和最严重的并发症

- 艾滋病的治疗只限于治疗复杂的感染和肿瘤

何　晨　何妙侠